Living with Multiple Myeloma

Practical advice from a fellow cancer survivor for myeloma patients, their family and friends

2012 Edition

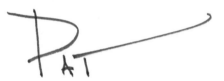

Pat Killingsworth

Red Fox Trail Press

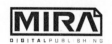
DIGITAL PUBLISHING

Published by Red Fox Trail Press
Info@RedFoxTrailPress.Com

Printed in the United States of America

ISBN 978-0-578-00339-9

Edited by Julie Ward
About the Editor:
Julie L.R. Ward earned her B.A., *magna cum laude,* in Biology with Education at St. Olaf
College, and her J.D., with honors, at the University of Minnesota Law School.
As editor, Julie draws from personal experience in a variety of fields including law and
public policy, insurance and finances, biology and related science, education and youth
work.
She may be reached at Julie.Ward@Centurytel.net

Copy design by Cathy Wimmer
Cover design by Mira Digital Publishing Formatted by The Copy
Shop - St. Croix Falls, Wisconsin_copyscf@centurytel.net
Website design and support by The Bit Works – Taylors Falls, Minnesota
info@thebitworks.com

Special Thanks

I would like to extend my heartfelt thanks to the Stillwater, Minnesota Multiple Myeloma Support Group members:

Barb Davis and Fatih Kinoglu
Gene and Eunice Early
Dan Faas
Kathie and John Gegen
Ardy and Peter Germann
Tom and Nancy Hansen
Alice and Roy Hallgren
Joyce and Dave Jenson
Steven Joachim
Pattie Killingsworth
Gene Kruschek
Gerry Landry and Annie Modesitt
Loren and Joan Liedl
Sharon Quast
Stacy Roher
Iwona Srienc
Bev Scully
Sue Shandley
Karl and Lorraine Vollstedt
Karen Wong and Tom Hayes
Don and Ardis Wright

Words cannot express how much your friendship and support have meant to me since I was first diagnosed in April, 2007. This book is dedicated to you.

Contents

Introduction

Why read a book like *Living with Multiple Myeloma*? So you or someone you know with multiple myeloma can take comfort in realizing there is hope. So you can learn from my or my medical team's mistakes–and realize you are not alone!

Multiple myeloma therapy options are changing so rapidly it has become difficult to keep up. After the dust settled following my initial diagnosis and treatment, I began to research myeloma therapy and nutrition in bookstores–a logical place to start for a middle-aged, former teacher who had relied on books as a primary information source over the years. But that didn't help. The books I could find had copyrights four, five or six years old. As I soon learned, that could be a lifetime in the world of multiple myeloma research.

I wanted to learn more about my cancer from a patient's perspective, so I started reading myeloma patient Websites. But these sites tended to be mostly emotional, with very little medical perspective. I wanted to know who these people were, but only enough about them to help me understand their frame of reference. I was more interested in why they had made their therapy decisions and what their treatments were like, not how their eight year old daughter was doing, or why Aunt Mabel could only come visit on Tuesdays.

I did eventually find a few bloggers who had interesting, informative sites. Even so, their content tended to lack focus. After all, these weren't professional writers who were thinking about the reader's needs. No, these patients were concentrating on their own medical and emotional challenges–their pacing and writing style varied from week-to-week and month-to-month, as the author's medical condition would ebb and flow.

The bottom line: There was no one source addressing the questions I needed answered. That is why my wife and caregiver, Pattie, and I started our two daily Websites: www.HelpWithCancer.org and www.MultipleMyelomaBlog.com. There you can find current information about the latest trends affecting myeloma patients, their caregivers and families, along with a number of helpful links to other myeloma Websites.

There is even a My Cancer Store, where you can

purchase recommended books about cancer, spirituality and nutrition at discounted prices.

Had I known more about multiple myeloma, and my therapy options in the beginning, I may have made better choices. I could have avoided several mistakes, made by my doctors, that have since had a negative effect on my long term quality of life.

That is why I wrote this book and update it every year. To try and help you organize your thoughts and focus on your important new life that lies ahead! I take this responsibility very seriously! Health permitting, I will update this book each and every year.

I have written a second book, *Stem Cell Transplants from a Patient's Perspective*, which addresses questions multiple myeloma patients and caregivers may have about stem cell transplants.

Living with multiple myeloma is truly one of life's ultimate challenges! I wish you, your friends and family all the best as you begin your new life's journey.

Fourteen Months

  Fourteen months ago I was diagnosed with Stage Two multiple myeloma. Has it only been fourteen months? It feels like a lifetime ago!

  I have been through so much in fourteen months! Large doses of radiation up and down my spine that left me sick, weak and disoriented. Heavy use of a potent steroid, dexamethasone, that caused nightly insomnia and my muscles to waste away. A pulmonary embolus left me hospitalized for five days and on oxygen for the next three weeks. An allergic reaction to a blood thinner that caused dangerously high fever and muscle aches. Monthly IV's. Oral chemotherapy. Constipation. Hemorrhoids. Low blood counts. Chills. A racing and elevated pulse rate.

A double hernia that presented itself after I lost eighteen pounds of muscle mass, in less than a month, caused by extreme radiation and steroid therapy. An affliction known as "chemo brain," which is the loss of short term memory resulting from chemotherapy. A scheduled six day visit to the Mayo Clinic to have my stem cells harvested for a future bone marrow transplant which actually took fifteen days to complete. A return visit to Mayo to have both hernias repaired. Surgically implanted catheters that would later become infected and need to be removed. CT scans. Full body x-rays. Labs. Pain meds. Antibiotics. Disintegrating vertebrae and compression fractures that left me almost two inches shorter than when I started. Oozing lesions in and around my spine. Large portions of rib bone weakened or missing. Bone marrow biopsies, both sedated and non sedated. Low blood counts. Anemia. Chills.

STOP! How did this happen? I am a fifty two year old male who was always in excellent health. A teacher and coach. A health club owner. A runner and ski instructor. But now I have cancer. A type of cancer that is usually reserved for those over the age of sixty-five.

Multiple myeloma is a cancer of the bone marrow. Specifically, the blood plasma that create white blood cells. When too many plasma cells are present in the bone marrow it can lead to decalcification of the bone, which can cause kidney failure as your kidneys clog and break down. Sometimes lesions (soft tissue tumors) form inside or outside the bones. My bones were slowly weakening and wasting away for years and I didn't even know it!

Fourteen months later and things are looking up! My weight is back to normal. Thanks to a daily exercise program, most of my muscle mass has returned. My body is tolerating monthly chemotherapy well and the insurance company is cooperating and paying for my treatment. Now, much of the time I feel good.

How did I get here and what do I do now? Hopefully, following my journey over the last fourteen months will help you, your family and friends adjust to living a life with multiple myeloma.

The Shower

My back was stiffer than normal. For almost one year I had been experiencing pain in my knees, ribs and back. My wife Pattie and I live in a beautiful area along the St Croix River that runs between Wisconsin and Minnesota, about an hour northeast of the Twin Cities. Woods, meadows, majestic views, and ticks— as in wood and deer ticks that can infect you or your pets with a dangerous assortment of bacterial infections.

Pattie and I have always been very athletic and active, spending a great deal of time outdoors, hiking and running our dogs through the many scenic parks in our area. But, especially in the spring, the ticks can be thick and, in my case, dangerous. Each of the previous two springs I had been infected with Lyme disease. Antibiotics helped, but often there were residual symptoms exactly like I was experiencing. I was having trouble walking up stairs and running or working out.

There was no detectable reason for my bone pain. I did manage to convince my family doctor after one of my now monthly examinations to give me an extended course of antibiotics. I had been reading about Lyme's. The number one complaint by patients and doctors in the know was antibiotics were often not used liberally enough to treat the disease.

Worth a try, but the antibiotics didn't seem to be helping. On this particular cold, damp Saturday morning in March, I was having an especially tough time getting started. My routine was simple: Take two ibuprofen with some Diet Coke (I don't drink coffee) and hobble to the shower. The hot water always felt good and helped get my joints and muscles moving again.

My lower back had been especially sore and stiff lately. Time for the chiropractor to "body slam" me again to loosen up my hip joints, so I could continue my sixty hour a week job as a Realtor at ERA Muske Company in St. Croix Falls, Wisconsin. Pattie and I had been listing and selling real estate since we moved to the area four years earlier. We both worked long hours. We were also both very active. Hiking, running with our dogs and swimming. Work hard, play hard and have fun had always been my motto. But my chronic pain was making it difficult for me to work or play. Visiting the chiropractor often helped, allowing me to do my job and hopefully enjoy some down time on weekends.

I suppose you could argue that I was in denial, that my deteriorating physical condition was a warning sign of something serious. But I wasn't too concerned. I was too busy, too caught up with day-to-day responsibilities and events to pay much attention. And, after all, I had been seeing my doctor regularly.

Still, my ribs had also been bothering me, especially on my right side. Had I pulled something working out? Odd my muscles were so slow to heal. Was it chronic Lyme disease?

All I know is, as I braced myself to sneeze that Saturday in the shower, my whole life changed. My left hand braced my ribs. My right hand braced my lower back. The force of the sneeze fractured my T-12 vertebra and the pain knocked me to my knees with such force that I almost passed out! It took me five minutes to turn off the water in the shower and somehow stand, bent and broken, leaning against the shower wall. I screamed in pain and for my wife to help, but she was downstairs feeding the dogs and did not hear me. I alternated between suffering silently and calling out to her for nearly fifteen minutes. Wet, cold and paralyzed with muscle spasms, I managed to drag myself to the sink and wait for her to hear my pleas for help. It took me 30 minutes to make it 20 feet into the bedroom where I sneezed again, throwing me against the wall as if shot with a gun!

Pattie had scheduled a real estate showing that morning and couldn't reach the buyers to cancel, so she called our licensed real estate assistant, Michele, to stop by the house and hopefully help me get into bed. (Is that part of any professional assistant's job description?) A good friend with a number of medical issues herself, Michele was more than happy to help. Pattie was able to get me into a robe before she left. Michele then carefully and deliberately eased me into bed. She thoughtfully gave me one of her Vicodin tablets, which helped! As long as I didn't move, laugh, cough or sneeze, the pain was manageable.

I spent most of the next week in bed. The following Saturday, I was going to try and show houses again, but the muscle spasms were so bad that I couldn't even make it into the emergency room to get more pain meds prescribed! Five phone calls by a very persuasive and determined wife netted me enough muscle relaxants to hold me over until I could get in and see a doctor on Monday.

My initial x-rays showed nothing wrong. On a second attempt, the physician on call at Osceola Medical Center noticed a small, possible hairline fracture of my T-12 vertebra. He prescribed bed rest and more pain meds. The muscle spasms slowly began to subside and, over the next few weeks, I was able to return to work.

The Moment

My chiropractor, Dr. Dwayne Truhlsen, had been pushing my insurance company to pay for an MRI for months. Now, with the help of my family doctor, Carrie Smith, at Osceola Medical Center, my insurance company agreed to allow the MRI which I had done at a specialty bone clinic in St Paul, Minnesota. The next day Dwayne called me. He asked if I could stop by after hours and discuss my results. He wouldn't give me any details over the phone, so I immediately thought the worst. Was it a disc? Arthritis? Another fracture?

April 3rd, 2007, 5:40 p.m. As I walked into Dwayne's darkened office he seemed visibly upset. Pattie and I sat down and faced an uncomfortable silence as Dr. Truhlsen tried to compose himself. I looked at Pattie, and she back at me. What was going on? Dr. Truhlsen was a young, strong, ambitious chiropractor with several offices in the area. He was building a new clinic, and we often talked about growth in the area and real estate. I appreciated his work ethic and enlightened approach to holistic medicine.

"Pat, I think that you have bone cancer." His eyes were red and teary. This was THE MOMENT. My wife is a two time cancer survivor. I spent years watching her endure surgeries and chemotherapy. I always wondered how it would feel to hear those words, to experience THE MOMENT. How would I react? How would it feel? Several times over the past six months I told Pattie that I believed there was something seriously wrong with me. I could sense it, feel it. I even joked it might be cancer. What was wrong with me?

But to hear it from my chiropractor! "Dwayne, you aren't supposed to be telling me this! This doesn't make any sense!" My anger was palpable. I was totally unprepared! "Why do you think I have cancer?" Dr Truhlsen mumbled something about my MRI. Pattie and I sat stunned. I felt her hand on my back as we both attempted to keep our composure. "Pat, there is bone damage, there are tumors, lesions. Dr. Smith has agreed to see you before her scheduled appointments tomorrow morning in Osceola."

I never used a chiropractor before Dr. Truhlsen. I didn't quite buy into the idea, and was always concerned I would become dependent on the adjustments. But my back and hip pain had gone far beyond the lingering injury

14

from a junior high school track meet which had bothered me over the years. The pain had increased so much I had to try something— even a chiropractor— to keep me moving.

Dr. Truhlsen was always organized and assertive. He insisted on taking full spinal x-rays prior to starting our twice weekly sessions. At times these sessions seemed to help. Other times not so much. But a second set of x-rays several months after I started therapy seemed to show improvement.

Now, here we all sat together, silently, in his empty office. Again Dwayne spoke. "Pat, I don't understand, I'm so sorry... The x-rays don't show any damage. No evidence of anything that I don't see every day." He clutched my films in both hands as if to suggest we look again to see what had been missed. But then he set the file down and slumped back in his chair, eyes red and hands trembling.

How ironic! My chiropractor had found what several extensive physical examinations the year before and a number of recent tests had not identified. I had cancer.

This Can't Be Good!

Dr. Kari Smith was the doctor on call when I first had trouble with Lyme disease the year before. You know you are getting old when your physician is young enough to be your daughter! But I was impressed by her systematic approach to medical problems. A good listener with a degree from the University of Minnesota – Duluth, Kari seemed open to suggestion and would cite recent medical studies to back her opinions.

Being self-employed, I had avoided the obligatory yearly physical examinations for financial reasons. Prior to my first bout of Lyme's, I had not had a physical for more than ten years. But after my fiftieth birthday and the subsequent Lyme Disease diagnosis, I decided to have a full physical examination.

In January 2006, Kari gave me a full medical exam. The Lyme's seemed to be gone, but I had some soreness in my ribs, knees, hips and back. Dr. Smith could find nothing wrong. Everything was fine! Blood work was good. Heart rate and blood pressure good. My PSA (a blood test to identify prostate cancer) was normal. My cholesterol was a bit high, but I hadn't been exercising as much as usual because of my aches and pains, so we decided to revisit that in about six months.

By summer my pain was a real problem. I had always been a runner but now I could barely run one mile without severe pain in my knees. I had also always been a golfer. While playing golf with my father in July, for the first time in my memory, I couldn't finish eighteen holes of golf, even riding in a cart. My mother suggested I visit a physical therapist friend that lived across the street from their home in Rockford, Illinois, where I was visiting. Amazingly, her friend, Jude, agreed to stop over after dinner. She gave me an impromptu therapy session in my parents' bedroom to try and loosen up my hip joints, back and shoulders. I'm not sure it helped, but I appreciated her effort!

After I returned home, Dr. Smith tested me a second time for Lyme disease. The test was inconclusive. No matter. One month later I was back in her office with a high fever and new tick bite on my back. The large, classic "bulls eye" rash surrounding the site was so well defined a number of doctors and nurses paraded through the exam room to view the spectacle.

I had been pushing Kari to prescribe some additional antibiotics even before the most recent bite, to see if it would help my deteriorating condition. Now I didn't need to lobby any longer. I left her office with a script for six more weeks of Doxcycline that cleared up the fever and rash almost immediately, but was not much help for my other symptoms.

All of that seemed like ancient history as Pattie and I drove to Osceola early the next morning. The clinic had just opened. I sat in Dr Smith's office waiting, wanting, needing to hear details about my condition. Kari entered the room with her nurse and assistant, Nancy, and sat facing me on a stool in front of the examination table. As she began to explain my situation, she, too, began to tear up, just as Dr. Truhlsen had done the evening before. She paused. I looked back at Pattie who was sitting to my right and remarked "This can't be good!" First Dwayne and now Kari. My immediate reaction was to comfort her. "This must be hard for you, Dr. Smith! What did you find? What can we do?" I remember also wryly conceding she had been right all along. My pain was not residual Lyme disease after all! A few moments later, she finished explaining she believed I had a type of cancer called multiple myeloma. How will we know for sure? "We have scheduled you for a bone marrow biopsy at Fairview Hospital in Minnesota. Tomorrow, ten a.m."

Biopsies

How do I best describe a bone marrow biopsy? Easy! Imagine someone bearing down on your lower back with all their weight using a corkscrew!

There are two types of bone marrow biopsies, sedated and non-sedated. I know several patients that don't seem to mind undergoing a non sedated biopsy. But if anything goes wrong, you will never get a non-sedated bone marrow biopsy again!

Of course, you usually need to undergo a procedure before you know any better. The area of choice for a bone marrow biopsy is most often in the lower back. I think physicians choose that particular spot because, since you are lying face down, you can't watch what is about to go down or hit the surgical tech as he starts to twist the coring tool slowly into the bone! Trust me, Novocain doesn't help!

But by the time that is made clear, it is too late. The twisting and pushing has begun, and all you can do is try to lie still while the nurses get a good look at your naked backside.

I will admit I have never been a fan of needles. Who is? But when you're stunned and facing your own mortality, you suck it up and tell yourself you have to do whatever it takes to get a handle on this thing! I actually thought I was enduring things quite well. But what should have been a two or three minute procedure was taking much longer. With tears in my eyes from the pressure and pain, I squeezed my nurse's hand harder and harder as the doctor stood on his toes to get more leverage. "Man, you have hard bones!" the doctor exclaimed, sounding frustrated. I finally gasped "Maybe you need a sharper tool!" "Great idea!" said the doctor as he asked the second nurse to bring a replacement. Ouch! I was kidding! Like he couldn't have figured out that his instrument wasn't sharp enough before he began?

There were now two nurses in the room. As they both tried to reassure me about how experienced my doctor was, he started the procedure again. Less than ten minutes later, I was back in the waiting room and headed home. I guess he had needed a sharper tool!

Although my first biopsy was probably worse than normal, my experience was not unusual. Many other myeloma patients I talked with during the months following have shared similar experiences. It hurts!

Second and third sedated bone marrow biopsy at the Mayo Clinic in June and September were not unpleasant experiences. Except for the nurse in training who couldn't get my IV started the first time, both procedures went off without a hitch, with very little discomfort. When given a choice, you may decide to try a non-sedated biopsy. However, I recommend that you learn from my mistake and ask for a sedated biopsy instead—or try a new, third alternative called OnControl.

The OnControl bone marrow biopsy option features a mechanized bone marrow system. Developed by Vidacare Corporation, the OnControl Bone Marrow System uses a patented power driver and needle technology to collect bone marrow aspirate and core samples. First used commercially in the fall of 2009, this new process is said to be faster and far less painful than a manual, non-sedated bone marrow biopsy.

I have experienced OnControl and it was a big improvement. It was faster and less painful. Tracy Gunnels and her husband, David, share my enthusiasm about this new system. In March of 2010, Tracy wrote: "Even if you don't have difficult biopsies, this system is still a necessity. My husband, David, had increasingly bad experiences (hard bones) and this system only took two minutes vs. 45 minutes without it! Once, David's doctor had his foot on the wall pushing, while I was pushing his hip from the other side! We cannot emphasize enough the value of this new tool."

Ouch! Sounds like I wasn't the first patient with hard bones and a difficult, painful biopsy experience! I checked around and it sounds like the new OnControl system is covered by most health insurance carriers. My fellow multiple myeloma patients may want to consider using OnControl. I have included contact information in the Information and Resource section at the end of this book.

Later that week, we received a disturbing phone call. I needed to return for an additional, second type of biopsy. This time the doctors would be biopsying one of the many tumors on my spine.

This was a surgical biopsy. I was unconscious and under general anesthesia for about thirty minutes. When I awoke in the recovery room the first face I saw was that of Mike Muske, my real estate broker and owner of ERA Muske Company. Still a bit disoriented, I wondered why was Mike here? How did he even know about my surgery? Mike was accompanied by one of our fellow agents Todd Kohs. I had only met Todd once, but I knew he had survived serious brain surgery several years before and was, himself, a cancer survivor.

I can't remember a time in my life when I was more surprised or touched. You see, Pattie and I had only recently switched real estate companies and joined the ERA Muske team. I knew Mike fairly well through contract negotiations, but he was a very busy guy. Mike owned eight real estate offices and managed hundreds of agents. But there he stood by my bedside, along with Todd and Pattie. I was moved, but also forced to face reality. Somehow the word was out. Knowing others knew about my condition seemed to make it more real. Pat was in trouble and needed help. Pat had cancer.

No! Don't Get Up!

Fairview Hospital is a large, regional medical center with a number of smaller branches in rural communities. The branch in Wyoming, Minnesota featured a state of the art radiation therapy unit. Located about thirty minutes north of St. Paul, Wyoming is a small bedroom community just beyond the suburbs, and twenty-five miles from my home across the river in St Croix Falls. Looking back on it now, I was fortunate to have such a highly rated facility so close to home. I wouldn't fully appreciate that fact until later, when following radiation therapy, those twenty-five mile car rides started to feel like forever!

It was a sunny, cool, April Wednesday in Minnesota. Pattie dropped me off in front of the Radiation Therapy

Department at Fairview. As we waited to meet my new doctor, we reflected upon the last four days. Was this all real? I hadn't called my parents in Rockford, Illinois until the second day after I had met Dr. Smith. My father, Ted, was a retired attorney who moved to Rockford from Evanston, Illinois, with his second wife, Jean, the year I began college at the University of Wisconsin. Like many families, ours had been affected deeply by cancer. His first wife, my mother Jeannie, died of lung cancer. Years later my father was diagnosed and treated successfully for prostate cancer. And, of course, my wife was a two time cancer survivor as well. Making the call to my family was one of the hardest things I ever had to do. On one hand, I needed and appreciated their support. But I knew how upsetting this would be for my aging father, considering our past history with the disease.

My parents reacted as I knew they would. Strong, supportive, positive. "Remember how well things turned out for Pattie and your father?" my mother said. "How can we help?" There was a long pause. "What can we do? Don't worry about the money! We will do whatever it takes to beat this thing!" The conversation went well, but my father was mostly silent as he listened on the other line. I could tell he was deeply upset.

My thoughts jerked back to the present as Dr. Xin Wang entered the room. A competent radiation oncologist, Dr. Wang was a pleasant man of few words. But his first words that day were some of the most memorable of my life. As I stood to shake his hand, Dr. Wang quickly strode across the room toward me, placed his hands firmly on my shoulders and blurted out, "No! Don't get up!" I sat back down, stunned and confused. "We don't want you to injure yourself. You must protect your spinal cord!" Dr Wang's Asian accent was thick, but his message was clear. He feared for my life!

Dazed, I don't remember much about the next ten minutes spent with Dr. Wang. But I remember vividly the films from my MRI, which he and his nurse, Joan, showed us slice by slice on the monitor in his office. Joan squeezed my shoulder in an attempt to reassure me as we all watched the small screen at the doctor's work station in disbelief. There were tumor-like masses called lesions oozing out between a number of my vertebrae. I was missing several inches of rib on both sides of my torso, replaced by a dark, gray, sponge like material. There were clearly visible holes in my right scapula, golf ball sized holes in my right pelvis and femur, and smaller holes in other bones. But more ominous were the large areas of missing bone in a number of my vertebra. In several sections, as much as one half of the bone had been replaced by the gray lesions that looked eerily similar to some amoeba-like alien creature from a sci-fi movie like *The Blob* or *Invasion of the Body Snatchers!*

The area that had sustained the most damage was in my lower and middle back, the same area where I had fractured my vertebra when I sneezed in the shower several weeks earlier.

Can you imagine how Pattie and I felt? The pain and muscle spasms from my vertebral fracture had been

27

excruciating and intense. Hearing about my cancer from Dr. Truhlsen had been difficult and surreal. But this! To see your own skeletal structure deteriorating before your very eyes!

I watched with horrified fascination as Dr. Wang finished explaining how and where he would radiate my spine. So as not to subject me to overly toxic levels of radiation, Dr. Wang decided to specifically hit the base of my neck and lower back from a number of different angles, targeting where my lesions were most prominent. The purpose of the radiation was to shrink the size and number of lesions, as well as kill cancer cells in the surrounding bone marrow. At the same time, I would start a daily regimen of steroid therapy designed to shrink the inflammation and ease the pain.

I regained my composure while watching the conclusion of Dr. Wang's diagnostic and treatment plan. Somehow getting caught up in the details of our plan of attack helped me focus on the task at hand. My treatment regimen would begin on Friday.

Trying to Work

I mentioned previously my wife and I are Realtors. The real estate market had not yet crashed in early 2006, but it was headed in the wrong direction. Realtors are paid by commission, not salary. If you don't work, you don't get paid! Throughout the muscle spasms and pain I tried to work. As soon as I was physically able (and often when I really wasn't!) I headed to the office or to showings. There were days when I could barely get out of my car in the parking lot. The four steps up to our offices became a daily challenge. It felt like I was climbing a mountain to get inside!

Fortunately, my wife helped pick up the slack and took care of many of the daily duties I handled previously: attending closings, training sales associates and completing listing paperwork. Pattie is amazing! A year earlier, she moved her infirmed mother to St. Croix Falls in order to help with her assisted living care. Also, although we never had children (Pattie's first surgery at age thirty-four ended any chance of that) we both were active in animal rescue. Up to twelve four-legged "kids" inhabited our hilltop home. You can imagine the time and energy Pattie needed to care for our rescued dogs and cats, not to mention the burden of cleaning the floors, upholstery and yard!

So let's add this all up. My wife was responsible for caring for her elderly mother, maintaining our active home on six acres, taking care of me and my deteriorating health, selling homes and, at times, handling much of my 60 hour workload as well. In her spare time, she tried to run, swim and exercise the animals. Did I mention our rescued canines were all former sled dogs that, unless exercised regularly, began to eat our furniture?

I want to stop here and stress although Pattie would, on occasion, allow her fatigue and frustration to show, it was never directed at me. She didn't have to imagine what I was going through. Pattie had been there! Her genuine concern about my health and well-being should be legendary. Her face would light up when the doctor or I shared any good news. If I felt better or if my blood work improved, Pattie was happy for me. Or if I could get up to go to the bathroom without assistance, when I hadn't been able to in the past, Pattie was sincerely excited for me. She never pushed, never complained. I felt her love all day, each and every day. I will never forget that!

The first day I tried to return to the office following my vertebral fracture and diagnosis, I experienced a narcotics overdose. I had been taking ibuprofen and Vicodin for the pain and muscle spasms. In an attempt to improve my pain management, Dr. Wang prescribed a Fentanyl patch. I always felt I was sensitive to medications in general. This was a perfect example of just how true that was!

I applied a standard sized Fentanyl patch to my upper arm after I was up and showered. Pattie dropped me off at the office and left to show some homes that morning. Within fifteen minutes after I applied the patch, I was so sick and disoriented that I asked Barb, a new, young agent in our office, if I could lie down in her car! She helped me out to her vehicle and I spent the next two hours, passenger seat reclined, windows wide open with the cold wind blowing in, trying to recover. After Pattie returned, she waited until I felt I was ready, then drove me to the Osceola Medical Center for an injection of Narcan to help clear my bloodstream. I never used another Fentanyl patch again!

Several days later I returned to my office. I struggled up the four stairs at our front entrance and was greeted inside by Barb, our office secretary Jessie, my assistant Michele, and partner Bruce. They took me to an empty storage room near the rear of the building and opened the door. Barb and Michele had set up a full sized futon in the room, along with pillows, blankets, a small refrigerator and other "comforts of home."

How thoughtful everyone had been! I then learned Barb and my friend, Deb Heichel from our ERA office in Osceola, had started a Caring Bridge website and blog for me, so I could keep a journal and hear from friends and family as my treatment progressed. The Caring Bridge site proved to be an inspirational revelation during my long and arduous recovery. But I am getting ahead of myself. That old saying is true; "It is always darkest before dawn!"

The Worst Six Weeks of My Life!

While all of this was going on, I was still recovering from my fractured vertebra. If you ever experienced severe back or muscle spasms you understand how painful and scary it could be! To cough or sneeze was excruciating! Worse still was the anticipation of the spasms. That in itself was sometimes paralyzing. A combination of Relaxol and Vicodin certainly helped. Of course, some people enjoy the high associated with such drugs. But as one who thinks twice about taking an aspirin, I was uncomfortable not being clear-headed.

It was Friday. Pattie helped me shower and dress. I was drugged and in pain. We made the thirty minute drive to Fairview Hospital to start my radiation treatments. There would be ten sessions starting that day and ending two weeks later. So far so good. But first would come the difficult task of carefully marking and actually tattooing my back and chest to assist the radiation techs in directing their massive robotic x-ray equipment. Now, normally an hour or two of this type of thing would only be inconvenient. But laying on that hard, cold table as my pain meds weakened, in uncomfortable positions only a gymnast would appreciate, didn't help the time go any faster!

The tedious process began at 1 p.m. By 4 p.m. we were ready to begin the first treatment. Fifteen more minutes and I would be out the door. Except that halfway through my radiation exposure the mechanism's software program inexplicably crashed. So there I lay for not one, not two, but three additional hours waiting for a repair tech to get things moving again. He could not get it done. We have all had to wait hours for the cable guy or refrigerator repairman to finally show up and get things fixed. That is inconvenient. This was maddening and unbelievable! By 7 p.m. everyone had determined the problem would not be solved that day. We would try again on Monday morning.

I have always been an athlete. I played and coached high school football. I believed I was a tough guy, able to play through pain. But the last month had certainly been a humbling experience!

Once the equipment was fixed and we settled into a daily routine, the first week of treatments was not so bad. "Don't worry," the radiation techs, Dr. Wang and other patients that I met throughout the week would say. The side effects of radiation therapy would be few and "tolerable."

I don't know if you have experienced this yet, but I never trust a doctor or nurse when they describe a procedure or side effects as tolerable. Tolerable to someone who isn't sick can mean something completely different than to the patient who is forced to endure the pain. To me, tolerable means the patient didn't die!

By the beginning of my second week, I was, unfortunately, proving them all wrong! The side effects were not tolerable, they were indescribably terrifying! Chronic fatigue was a common experience among radiation therapy patients. I knew because I asked. I met some very positive, brave patients in the waiting and locker room areas over the next few weeks. Some felt nothing. Some became progressively more tired as therapy continued. Prostate cancer patients often had bowel or bladder issues. Breast cancer patients seemed to have few, if any, side effects. A few patients I talked to experienced nausea and constipation. No one seemed to think my radiation therapy would be more than a minor inconvenience.

I'm not sure why the treatments hit me so hard. Maybe it was the large amount of radiation they used at multiple points up and down my spine. Maybe it was the combination of the radiation and my dexamethasone steroid therapy. It wasn't my narcotics use. I discontinued that as the steroids began to help with the pain and I became slightly nauseated and disoriented from the radiation.

By the end of my seventh treatment I was sick. Really sick. Pattie was forced to pull our vehicle over several times for me to recover enough to continue traveling. I tried drinking soda and eating pretzels on the way home but that didn't help. It only got worse. That weekend I could barely eat. The room was spinning. I didn't have the strength to get up but I felt like I couldn't stay still or lie down.

Our home is all on one level, but upstairs. We have a tuck-under garage and full basement with stairs leading up from the garage on the inside and a long set of stairs up to the front door outside. By my eighth or ninth treatment, it would take me ten minutes to climb the stairs. I couldn't focus on anything. I couldn't read or watch TV. Resting and convalescing can be a tolerable or even enjoyable experience. This was neither.

Worst of all, I couldn't focus my thoughts. Everything had happened so quickly! Pain, diagnosis, treatment. I hadn't had time to process it all. Looking back, I felt cheated. I needed that lost time to think. To read.

To get a handle on my treatment options and to learn more about my cancer. To think about our finances and future. To work through the five steps of mourning. In short, I hadn't had time to adjust; I hadn't had time to grieve.

That would all have to wait. I was trying to hang on minute by minute. I couldn't sleep or eat. I was experiencing horrible night sweats. When I could sleep the dreams were terrible nightmares about fighting a variety of villains and creatures. Often the dreams were more direct. I would dream about my fight with cancer. Lying in bed struggling to stay alive. Struggling to find help, to find hope. I would wake relieved. Was it all a dream? Night after night I would wake up, confused and disoriented, soaked in my sweat and sometimes blood.

I am not a big guy. Five foot eight inches tall and about one hundred sixty pounds. But in just over two weeks I lost over eighteen pounds, most of it muscle! Sick, tired, nauseated and emaciated, I somehow made it to the hospital for what I thought would be my final treatment on Friday. Remember the technical difficulties we experienced at my first marathon session several weeks before? The techs had only been able to complete one half of my treatment. As I politicked Dr. Wang to allow me to skip that last one half session, my spirits sank to an all-time low as he refused to budge. I would be forced to return Monday to make up that additional session.

Now under normal circumstances that would have been no big deal. What's another trip back to the hospital? Most nurses, fellow patients and Internet reading Pattie did about my therapy (remember that I couldn't read!) led us to believe I should start feeling better within a few days after the last session. In my current physical and mental state that three day delay to the start of my recovery time was devastating. Utterly devastating. I was so tired of being sick! This was the lowest point for me, physically and emotionally, since I was diagnosed. But as usual, Pattie's steady and constant support helped me to re-group and make it to my last treatment on Monday. I enthusiastically allowed Pattie to help me get into our vehicle for the last trip to Minnesota. One more visit!

Soon this would all be over and I could rest and focus. Now things would get better, right?

No, things did not get better. Despite drinking cases of high calorie shakes and trying to eat, even if I couldn't stand the taste or smell of any type of food, my weight dropped even further. Pattie shared with me how she made it through her chemo by eating mac and cheese and peanut butter. I humored her and tried to eat as much of the different foods that she would prepare as possible, but eating anything was a struggle.

I have never had trouble eating! I am usually hungry all the time. So the fact I wasn't interested in eating reinforced Pattie's concerns about my condition. Days later I was still sick. One week later still sick. Now, mid-May, I tried to sit on our deck in the sun, but could only hold myself up for five, maybe ten minutes. I forced myself to walk down the hill to get the mail. I kept trying to eat.

I was still having horrifying, exhausting nightmares. But about a week after my final treatment, I awoke and realized that I was repeating a battle every night that I didn't need to fight! I was safe, lying in my own bed. I wasn't dying, at least not right away. Instantaneously I felt my body relax. I could save my energy to fight the real battles that lie ahead. The nightmares never returned.

By the end of the second week following my last session at Fairview I finally improved enough to read for short periods of time or sit up and watch TV. I could now walk to the end of our block and back. The first time I made it all the way I raised my arms in triumph and yelled

"YES!" out loud. You would have thought I had just won a marathon!

But I was still having trouble sleeping. If I was lucky, I could sleep until five a.m. Often I would wake, only to toss and turn, as early as two a.m. I didn't know it at the time, but my daily doses of dexamethasone were causing my insomnia. The dex was most likely the major contributor to my night sweats and nightmares as well. This had one benefit. Since it was now possible for me to read and focus my thoughts, I soon figured out I could use this early morning time to reflect on my new lot in life. I would think about my situation, my condition, my treatment. I would read, pay bills, look over my medical reports and try to adjust to life after cancer.

Lance Armstrong

The first book that I read after I was diagnosed with cancer in April 2007 was Lance Armstrong's It's Not About the Bike. Big mistake! Armstrong's book was written with emotion and strength. It was about his successful fight against testicular cancer— a superhuman athlete battling an advanced form of cancer that was difficult, if not impossible, to treat. Fighting terrible odds and using toxic and extreme forms of chemotherapy, Armstrong defeated cancer with the same will and determination that he used to conquer the Alps in the Tour de France.

It's a great story that left me feeling lame and inadequate. I wasn't having radioactive isotopes and heavy metals pumped throughout my body in doses that would kill any normal human. I wasn't riding an exercise bike for an hour in my hospital room the day after surviving major brain surgery. Armstrong ate only free range chicken and organic broccoli; even his diet left me feeling like a wimp! Why was I so weak and so sick, when others experiencing radiation weren't? Why did I have a type of cancer that was most common in older people? After all, the average multiple myeloma patient is first diagnosed with the disease at age sixty-eight. I had just turned fifty-one.

Yet at the same time, Lance Armstrong's story did inspire me and fundamentally changed my way of thinking about cancer. Up to this point I had been in a daze, a trance. In my defense, part of that was drug induced! Still, why had I been so accepting of my situation and condition?

When I was sickest toward the end of my radiation and steroid treatments, I experienced, for the first time in my life, the acceptance of death. I was dizzy, disoriented, weak and in pain. Death didn't seem so intimidating. I could actually imagine letting go.

I was always a high energy, type "A" personality type of guy! A fighter who valued every minute of every day. Someone who loved life and couldn't understand those who would give up or end their own lives. What a waste, right? Cancer patients often write about the "fight." Cancer is an enemy to be conquered and defeated. Why didn't I feel this way? I was a very competitive person. Why wasn't I embracing this battle?

Up to this point I hadn't been fighting. I had been fatalistically accepting my condition, just trying to hang on, sleep walking through my treatment. Reading Lance

Armstrong's book helped me change that. It was time to become proactive. It was time to fight!

Mayo Clinic

The first step in my fight for survival was to learn more about my cancer. I was definitely "technically challenged," and I used a computer for my job as a Realtor reluctantly. E-mail, home searches, some marketing. But at least I was familiar with the Internet, and quickly learned more than I wanted to know about my disease. There was no cure. Although the average patient experienced some success initially by using a variety of chemotherapy regimens and, if possible, undergoing a bone marrow transplant, the life expectancy for a Stage Two multiple myeloma patient in May, 2007 was forty-three months.

I immediately located two exceptional multiple myeloma treatment centers with distinctly different treatment philosophies: The Myeloma Institute in Little

Rock, Arkansas and the Mayo Clinic in Rochester, Minnesota.

The reason for the Myeloma Institutes particular location became apparent when I learned that Wal-Mart founder Sam Walton had died of multiple myeloma in Arkansas. Mr. Walton left a large part of his fortune to establish a preeminent cancer center there, specializing in multiple myeloma treatment and research.

Oncologists in Little Rock are big fans of stem cell transplants. Doctors there developed a process using back to back transplants called tandem transplantation. This was cutting edge science in the late 1990's. It was hoped that these dual procedures might help extend the before mentioned forty-three month average lifespan of myeloma patients by a year or two. Some recipients had even been cured. But tandem transplants could be dangerous. Not only that, but some recent studies contradicted the Institute's claims that tandem transplantation was superior to using newly developed chemotherapy in conjunction with a single stem cell transplant.

Author's Note: I have since learned that the Myeloma Institute pioneered a treatment regimen called Total Therapy. I feature a lot of information about Total Therapy on my daily Website: www.MultipleMyelomaBlog.com. This controversial approach throws everything but the kitchen sink at newly diagnosed myeloma patients—cocktails of three, four and five drugs before and after tandem stem cell transplants. Docs there are getting some great, long term results, especially among younger, low risk patients. Some are even using the word "cure." But this treatment option is not for the faint of heart! It can be a hard, long road—up to five years of aggressive therapy. It can also be expensive—and some insurance plans won't cover it because it is considered experimental or out of network. Despite the risks, newly diagnosed patients may want to research Total Therapy.

The second nationally recognized treatment facility I researched was Mayo Clinic. Although Mayo had other hospitals located in Arizona and Florida, the primary facility was located in Rochester, Minnesota, just over two hours away from my home in St. Croix Falls. I learned doctors at Mayo perform over two hundred stem cell transplants each year—and Mayo seemed to feature a more balanced approach to treatment. There were a number of new cancer fighting drugs available to patients like myself, thanks to studies conducted there and at other institutions specializing in blood and lymphatic cancers.

How would I get started? The waiting list to see a specialist at Mayo was weeks long, and time was definitely not on my side! Did I know anyone who might know someone who could help me get a consult at Mayo? Do you believe in miracles?

Remember my new found friend and cancer survivor, Todd Kohs, at my bedside following my biopsy at Fairview Hosptial? The day after I felt well enough to begin researching my choices, Todd called me out of the blue on my cell phone. How was I feeling? What were my treatment options? Was there any way he could help? Before I could even bring up the Mayo Clinic, Todd suggested I try there. It turned out he had his brain surgery at Mayo. Todd wanted to help.

The next morning my wife's cell phone rang. On the line was Jerry Wollner, a retired administrator from Mayo and a friend of Todds. He had referred our case to Dr. Robert Kyle, who specialized in myeloma. Often called "the father of modern multiple myeloma research and treatment," Dr. Kyle was calling from his home. Calling us, now, today, on Pattie's cell phone! He listened carefully as I described my situation, diagnosis and treatment to date. Dr. Kyle was calm and reassuring. He said he could help. The next week I was headed to Rochester.

I was still not feeling well as Pattie and I packed up the SUV and began the drive to Rochester. My weight was still down. I was dizzy and weak.

While at Mayo I would undergo a number of tests. The first stop was for a blood draw. Nineteen vials of blood. The med tech joked that was as much blood as a woman, giving birth might be expected to lose—then she would get a transfusion! I wasn't laughing. Next, I was handed the large, plastic container for my twenty-four hour urine collection. How fun to visit a fast food restaurant with brown bag and jug in tow! I wondered if this was how the term "brown bagging it" got started?

Reading this in my first book draft, Pattie recalled a nice couple from the Upper Peninsula of Michigan we met at Mayo. The wife was also being treated for myeloma. Feeling pretty good and having several hours to kill, they snuck away to play nine holes of golf. The couple rented a golf cart and began to play. On the third hole, a course supervisor stopped to remind them "carryon's" or beverages of any type were not allowed on the course unless purchased from the bar. He had seen her brown bag, complete with jug, and assumed it was a consumable beverage!

On to x-ray for my full body series of films. They didn't do another MRI. But I did see a Mayo certified dentist for a set of teeth and jaw films, as well as x-rays of my head from several angles.

When you have multiple myeloma, doctors pay a lot of attention to your dental health. One of the first treatments you receive is a biophosphonate IV of either Aredia or Zometa. These medications are designed to strengthen your bones and work to shrink any lesions or tumors that may be present. Such lesions can be in the bone or, in my case, oozing out between the ribs or vertebrae. One of the possible side effects of these treatments is called "osteonecrosis of the jaw."

Any weakness of the jaw or dental issues such as a cracked filling or inflamed wisdom tooth increases the risk of this side effect. Symptoms can include tingling and loss of feeling in the jaw or mouth, pain and/or loss of integrity of the jaw bone. In other words, your jaw bone starts to die and can break down and disintegrate! This can be especially troublesome, since many of these unpleasant symptoms are irreversible.

At a time when any good news was a welcome diversion, it was reassuring when the dentist handling the consult emerged from the back offices with a smile and thumbs up sign. My x-rays looked great! No worries there.

Looking back, this didn't seem like a big deal. But in subsequent months I met a number of myeloma patients who suffered serious deterioration of their skull. Several also had large lesions there as well. A fellow multiple myeloma patient, Alice Hallgren, experienced irreversible necrosis of the jaw following IV treatments using the biophosphonate Zometa. I was fortunate not to have had any bone damage above my shoulders. Thank God for small blessings!

Now to the consultations. We met with a social worker who helped us apply for a grant through the Leukemia and Lymphoma Society. She also brought us up to speed on possible living arrangements for my future stay at Mayo, when I would undergo a stem cell transplant. Not "if" I had a transplant, but "when." (More on this later!) We also met with a spiritual counselor and several nurses who helped address our concerns.

Mayo Clinic is amazingly well organized. Prior to each visit you receive an hour by hour itinerary in the mail, complete with directions to each department. Also included are any testing restrictions or requirements that there might be, such as, "Don't eat any hard food after eight p.m. the day before you arrive."

The campus, as it is called, is quite impressive. Our first impression of the upper levels of the main building was that of being on the deck of a cruise ship. Beth Morgan, author of a popular myeloma related website, *Beth's Blog*, had a similar impression when she first arrived: "I had my first day of tests at the Mayo Clinic. First, let me say that I'm awe struck by the facility itself. Everywhere I've been has been clean and well-run. There's some real architectural beauty there as well. It's like the Disneyland of health care. I mean it. It's really nice! I don't want to name any names, but I've been in other places in which all I could think about was how icky and gross they are. You know what I mean. Those places where you're scared to sit in the chairs in the waiting rooms because of those dark stains on the upholstery. Not to mention the big stains of questionable origin on the carpet. I usually feel contaminated when I'm there. This wasn't the case at the Mayo Clinic."

Although we never met, Beth and I were undergoing testing in Rochester at the same time that fateful May. We shared the same doctor and endured many of the same tests. I'm sure we passed each other several times in the halls, or sat next to each other in one of the waiting rooms. Beth from Southern Pines, North Carolina, and me from Wisconsin. Guess it is a small world when you are diagnosed with multiple myeloma!

A very small world. Five weeks after I learned I had cancer, another Realtor in our company, Karen Wong, was also diagnosed with multiple myeloma. Karen was a small, thin, energetic woman in her sixties. It was an interesting coincidence we were both diagnosed with the same type of cancer at the same time. But what was even more unusual was that Karen would have myeloma at all.

Multiple myeloma is more common in men than women. It is more common is African American men than white men. A woman of Asian descent is the least likely American to be diagnosed with this type of cancer.

I barely knew Karen. We did not work in the same office. We had only spoken once or twice at company meetings, at our company headquarters in Forest Lake. So you can imagine my surprise when I learned Karen was also going to Mayo Clinic for tests that same week. She called me my second day there. Did I feel well enough to meet her for lunch?

As we talked, I noticed a woman in a stylish sweat suit also speaking on her cell phone a few tables away. It was Karen! I laughed and walked over to her table, cell phone in hand. She was with her husband, Tom Hayes. Pattie and I gladly joined them for lunch.

Karen was to be undergoing many of the same tests I began the previous morning. Like me, she was surprised by her diagnosis. Like me, Todd Kohls from Forest Lake had helped get her foot in the door at Mayo Clinic. Fortunately for Karen, she did not need the debilitating radiation therapy I had undergone the past month. Unfortunately for Karen, she learned surgery would be required to stabilize the weakened bones in her legs and hips.

You can guess we bonded immediately. Karen and I spent the next year sharing our experiences and helping each other cope with our new, difficult reality. We remain good friends today.

Located in Minnesota, Rochester can get cold! To help overcome this unpleasant obstacle for its many visitors from around the world, all of the medical buildings are connected by a series of tunnels and glass walkways crisscrossing the campus above and below ground. An entire underground city has developed, including a variety of restaurants, shops and impressive atriums, decorated with colorful murals and expensive works of art. It leaves you with a very calming, even spiritual feeling palpable from the moment you arrive.

One of the many features down below is a series of patient friendly lounge and break areas. Several of these rooms are kept dark and are filled with beds and recliners so that patients can rest between appointments. I took advantage of these areas a number of times, as I had little stamina and remained dizzy and weak. Pattie would check our e-mail in one of the neighboring computer rooms while I rested and tried to sleep. They think of everything at Mayo!

My final meeting was with oncologist Dr. Steven Zeldenrust. By now, I was exhausted and having trouble focusing. Pattie and I waited for him nervously in his small but well-appointed office. I felt weak and agitated. I couldn't sit still, so I paced while I read his diplomas and framed awards on the wall. A graduate of the University of Indiana, Dr. Zeldenrust was a young, personable guy who was reassuring and easy to talk with.

All of our news was good! My cancer was not progressing quickly but, as we knew, the damage was great. Dr. Zeldenrust felt that I had multiple myeloma for a number of years. Much of the bone damage would repair itself with time as long as we could keep my cancer under control. He was missing one important piece of information concerning my genetic predisposition to the disease. Apparently, a number of myeloma patients are missing a chromosome, making it difficult to treat. He would call me the following week and let me know if I was missing the all-important thirteenth chromosome. But in the meantime, my blood work had improved with the combination of steroid and radiation therapy, and he was pleased. Dr. Zeldenrust felt I was a prime candidate for a transplant and that we should schedule one as soon as possible.

As soon as possible meant two things. First, I would need to take a new and very expensive form of oral chemotherapy, called Revlimid, for at least three months, along with even larger doses of dexamethasone. Second, Mayo had a very tightly scheduled transplant waiting list. Dr. Zeldenrust would see what he could do.

Prognosis and Survival Rates

The good news about being diagnosed so suddenly and dramatically is I have never felt I was denied anything. I had always been an active runner and athlete. Basketball, tennis, golf, skiing. I continued to participate in regular sports and physical activities until the pain from unknown causes forced me to slow down as I neared my fiftieth birthday. I didn't write about it before, but Doctors Truhlsen, Smith and Wang had all been quietly pessimistic about my prognosis. Following my fateful MRI and early treatment and weight loss that left me sick and emaciated, any activity or function that became possible was a blessing. From being nauseous and disoriented to being able to walk and function day to day, every improvement was a victory. It wasn't until after my first meeting with Dr. Zeldenrust that I began to feel real hope.

Everything happened too fast. I never focused on the things that I could not do or was denied, but on the number of activities that I could complete. So even though it is difficult and painful for me to run to this day because of damage to the lower cervical area of my spine (just below my neck), I walk, bike and swim instead. I could ski, but an unexpected fall might lead to fracture in any number of places where the cancer has weakened my bones. I could golf, but the disease has left me so shaky it would be difficult to putt well and painful to strike the hard ground with my club. Golf was very time consuming. By giving up the game, I have learned to use that time for things I value more. Time with family and friends. Working on the house. Taking a long, leisurely walk with the dogs and my wife. Writing this book!

I spoke with Dr Zeldenrust following my trip to Mayo. More great news! I was not missing the all-important thirteenth chromosome, making me a prime candidate for a bone marrow transplant. In my mind, the even better news was my cancer was progressing very slowly. Not only that, but the radiation and dexamethasone regimen had been surprisingly effective! The cancer was responding to treatment.

I was also starting to feel better. I could think clearly again. But be careful what you wish for! With clarity came questions, lots of questions. Now that we knew the cancer was responding, what was my prognosis? Would the damage to my ribs and bones stop? Could the damage be reversed and repaired? What were my treatment options? In short, what was next?

It was time to call the doctor. Dr. Zeldenrust listened patiently to all of my questions. I must say I was impressed and touched. Here was a busy oncologist at the renowned Mayo Clinic, addressing each question one by one with sensitivity and compassion. During the course of my forty minute phone call I learned my multiple myeloma was in Stage Two.

Most cancer is diagnosed in stages. How far your particular cancer has progressed and where that fits on the appropriate scale helps physicians determine a patient's initial prognosis. I highly recommend newly diagnosed multiple myeloma patients read the book, *100 Questions & Answers About Myeloma,* written collaboratively by Asad Bashey, Raft Abonour and James Huston. This book discusses multiple myeloma in a straightforward fashion that is easy for patients and their families to read and understand.

100 Questions & Answers About Myeloma provides a detailed summary of the Durie-Salmon staging system for multiple myeloma. First developed in 1975, this commonly used analysis uses three stages to define a patient's condition.

In Stage One, a relatively small number of myeloma cells are present throughout the body. A patient will have no apparent symptoms. Measurable amounts of monoclonal protein found in the blood or urine are still low. Monoclonal protein is a type of antibody or immunoglobulin produced by myeloma cells. It is used as a marker to help monitor the progress of the cancer. A healthy person has little or no monoclonal protein in their blood or urine.

A patient in Stage Two will have much higher levels of monoclonal protein present and also exhibit some initial symptoms or damage caused by the disease.

A Stage Three diagnosis means a patient has a large number of myeloma cells present throughout the body. In addition, a patient may be anemic, with high blood calcium levels, multiple lytic bone lesions and/or have high levels of monoclonal protein in their blood or urine. Lytic lesions are thinning areas of the bone that look like holes on an x-ray. I had a number of these "holes" in my bones!

Since multiple myeloma symptoms and progression vary so widely from patient to patient, my impression is it is can be a very difficult cancer to stage. In most cancers, where you fall on the staging time line makes a significant difference for your overall survival rate. Myeloma staging may be less relevant when used to predict a patient's life expectancy; in multiple myeloma, a patient's stage when diagnosed is often not as important as how well the cancer initially responds to treatment.

In my case, my monoclonal protein level was high, but not off the charts. I had several lytic lesions with substantial bone damage. But apparently my cancer had been progressing so slowly I had normal calcium levels in my bloodstream. Controlling calcium in your blood is of utmost importance. It is elevated calcium levels that causes damage to a patient's kidneys, liver and other organs. On the Durie-Salmon staging system, I was clearly Stage Two, not Stage Three, because most of my blood work was normal. Using several different staging methods, Dr. Zeldenrust classified me as IPI Stage One and Durie-Salmon Stage Two. The fact my cancer had already responded well to treatment was encouraging. The heavy radiation and dexamethasone dosing had already cut my monoclonal protein levels in half. We would start chemotherapy right away for a period of three or four months in an effort to destroy as many myeloma cells as possible prior to my transplant. This would require walking a fine line; too many remaining cancer cells might hurt the long term outcome of my transplant. But prolonged chemotherapy could damage healthy stem cells that would need to be harvested and used later to replenish my bone marrow after it had been destroyed during the transplantation process.

Dr. Zeldenrust informed me that Mayo had been using a drug called Revlimid which, up to this point, was only approved for use in relapsed myeloma patients. It had shown great promise for use in pre-transplant patients. Revlimid (lenalidomide) was effective in reducing the number of cancer cells in the bone marrow without damaging the integrity of remaining cells needed later for transplant.

Oncologists had been using another chemotherapy agent, thalidomide, to do this. Dr. Zeldenrust shared with me that Revlimid was an analog, or second generation, form of thalidomide. Apparently, Revlimid had far fewer side effects than thalidomide. But there might be a catch. The FDA had not yet formally approved Revlimid for first line treatment of multiple myeloma. Some insurance companies were refusing to reimburse patients for its cost when Revlimid was used this way. In that case, Dr. Zeldenrust would administer thalidomide as a substitute, because Revlimid was very expensive—close to seven thousand dollars a month!

But Dr. Zeldenrust assured me my Blue Cross/ Blue Shield insurance should cover the cost of this new drug, and we could schedule my transplant accordingly. Three months of chemo, with an extra week or two to deal with the insurance company, would put us into mid to late August. Dr. Zeldenrust's assistant would mail me an itinerary the next week.

I had read conflicting views on the Internet about the ability of my bones to repair themselves. Dr Zeldenrust recommended that I start using a biophosphonate called Aredia to help speed the process. This should help my bones recover. "There isn't any reason that, for as long as we can keep the cancer in check, your bones won't continue to heal." I later learned that would indeed be the case, with the exception of major damage such as missing ribs, severe compression fractures or large holes in my bones that might never totally fill in. He said I should start my monthly, three hour Aredia IV treatments immediately, continuing them for up to two years we work to stabilize my skeletal integrity.

Wow! We had a plan! But what was the goal? "As you know Pat, there is no cure for multiple myeloma. If all goes well with the transplant, you should be able to live one, two, maybe even three years without chemo or other types of invasive therapies." "But what then, Doctor?" I asked anxiously. "Well, when the cancer comes back we can try other types of chemotherapy or possibly even another transplant."

WHEN the cancer comes back! Not IF the cancer comes back. That was a sobering thought! My mind was racing through a whole new list of questions. How does someone die from multiple myeloma? Is it painful? How long do you live after you exhaust your medical options? Is there hope?

Dr Zeldenrust did his best to try and explain the time line. He told me the average Stage Two patient survives forty-three months. Having a transplant does not necessarily extend that number. It becomes a quality of life issue. Live relatively drug free for several years, or fight the disease daily using a combination of expensive medications with varying side effects, while the drugs and cancer wear you down. Eventually, your bones lose their integrity and begin to deteriorate. The high levels of calcium released into your bloodstream damage your kidneys and other organs and they, too, begin to fail. Most myeloma patients ultimately need dialysis. Their kidneys fail, then their liver.

"But doctor, some patients must live longer than three or four years!" I asked in a firm and determined way. "Of course they do! Forty-three months is an average. But Pat, only ten percent of our patients live ten years. It looks like you should do well, but there are no real predictors. Things are looking good for you so far, but this is a serious disease..." His voice trailed off. I appreciated his honesty and approach to our plan. I trusted him. But what are the side effects? How is the chemotherapy administered? Where will I be treated? Will I have to drive down to Mayo every week? Every month? By the time I formulated my next set of questions, Dr. Zeldenrust had reminded me to expect my August itinerary in the mail soon and we had said our goodbyes.

Author's Note: Don't despair my fellow multiple myeloma patients! The treatment landscape has changed for the better since the spring of 2007. A short three years later, life expectancy numbers are improving rapidly for all but the least fortunate among us. Exactly how much median life expectancy numbers have improved is open to interpretation. But few question that multiple myeloma patients are beginning to live longer with the help of new, novel therapies like Thalomid, Revlimid and Velcade.

With such a wide variety of therapy combinations being used across the country, it is hard to track patient progress with any certainty. Unfortunately, researchers don't yet know which drugs, or combination of drugs work best. Why? Results seem to vary greatly between patients. And, since so few patients using these new therapies are dying, it has become difficult to compile enough reliable data to do much more than guess how long a myeloma patient may live. How exciting is that!

Osceola Medical Center

Osceola is a historic river town located on the east bank of the St. Croix River in west central Wisconsin. Just close enough to the Twin Cities for some to consider it a bedroom community, Osceola's claim to fame is its scenic beauty and the long, clear span bridge that connects it to Minnesota.

There are only five bridges crossing the St Croix along a hundred mile stretch of river that divides Minnesota from Wisconsin. St. Croix Falls and Osceola lay right in the center of that span about eight miles apart.

Much too small to support a full-time oncologist, Osceola Medical Center contracts with Regions Hospital in St Paul to make some of its specialists available to patients in Osceola. That way, patients get the benefit of working with a qualified specialist without having to drive an hour and park in the Cities.

I met with Dr. Daniel Anderson for an initial consult at Regions Hospital in St. Paul. As I had recently learned, putting together my medical support team was one of the most important steps I would take along my journey towards recovery. I had a general practitioner or family doctor, Dr. Smith, in Osceola. My radiation oncologist, Dr. Wang would continue to be available should I need any further localized radiation treatments. Dr. Zeldenrust was my clinical oncologist at Mayo, specializing in the treatment of multiple myeloma. Dr. Anderson would become my medical or general oncologist and help monitor my progress. He would also be the one to prescribe my chemotherapy and other cancer related medications. Later I would be adding a nutritionist and other important members to my cancer fighting team as well.

I was very pleased after my first meeting with Dr. Anderson. He was young, personable and obviously very bright. He was also very positive in his approach and very receptive to working closely with the doctors at Mayo. He enthusiastically promised to consult with Dr. Zeldenrust before setting any new treatment protocol. I was also very happy to know that I could see Dr. Anderson monthly in Osceola and receive any of my medications and treatments locally.

I quickly discovered the oncology support staff in Osceola was excellent. Oncology nurses, Dody Lunde and Cathleen McGinnity, were both experienced and compassionate. There is something deeply reassuring about receiving treatment in familiar surroundings close to home. Dr. Anderson consulted with Dr. Zeldenrust at Mayo and determined the best combination of chemotherapy drugs for me to take would be the experimental Revlimid and the steroid I was already taking, dexamethasone. Dr. Anderson was more than willing to help me convince my insurance company to pay for this treatment option. Both Dr. Anderson and Dr. Zeldenrust believed I would have very little problem getting my treatment protocol approved. I felt we were making progress; as if I now had clinical support and Pattie and I weren't in this alone. I was beginning to feel better, my weight was slowly coming back and we had a plan of attack that had consistently shown positive results with a majority of other similarly diagnosed patients. Things would only get better, right?

Insurance and the International Myeloma Foundation

Most Realtors are self-employed sales agents working for a broker without any company provided benefits. Having spent years helping Pattie battle her cancers, I knew the importance of good insurance. Shortly after moving to the St. Croix River valley and becoming active again in real estate, I carefully shopped for a major medical insurance policy. Since I had never been a smoker or had cardiovascular or cancer related health issues in my past, I had a choice of a number of insurance companies and plans that might fit my needs. I eventually selected a Blue Cross/Blue Shield of Wisconsin plan with a large three thousand dollar deductible, but a broad range of coverages allowing me to see physicians on both sides of the river. I chose not to buy a prescription drug plan. In retrospect that would have been great to have, but my thinking at the time was I could pay for an occasional pain medication or antibiotic on my own and save the fifty dollar a month additional premium payment. That way I could also avoid dealing with drug co-pays and the headaches I associated with drug plans.

My insurance agent, Doug Willert, did have the foresight to anticipate any major drug expenditures would be covered by my major medical policy after I reached my deductible. Yes, it would have been nice to get some early help with some of my medications. But I reached my deductible so quickly during those early whirlwind days of diagnosis and treatment that the effects of my choice were insignificant. However, after learning how expensive my IV and chemotherapy drugs were, I must admit that I would have experienced a perverted pleasure paying for a seven thousand dollar drug with a ten or twenty dollar co-pay!

Did I say seven thousand dollars? That might be a bit of an exaggeration. Try sixty-eight hundred and change. That's right! One month's supply of twenty-one twenty-five mg Revlimid capsules costs over sixty-eight hundred dollars! But hey, they deliver the capsules right to your door by next day air so it must be worth it, right? Actually, yes, it is worth it if it works, and if you can afford to pay that much each month.

I was fortunate to have insurance. But what about someone who had pre-existing conditions (like my wife) or who couldn't afford insurance at all? I will revisit these and other insurance related issues later in the book. For now, I felt confident that my insurance was comprehensive and would be effective.

That was until I heard back from Blue Cross/Blue Shield of Wisconsin in a certified letter dated May 11th, 2007, denying Dr. Anderson's request to authorize payment and my subsequent treatment using Revlimid and dexamethasone.

Frustrated, upset and looking for answers, I called the International Myeloma Foundation's patient help line. It was after seven p.m. Central Standard Time, but the IMF was located in California so I thought it might be worth a try. A knowledgeable and reassuring voice on the other end of the line answered my questions about multiple myeloma, treatment options and their side effects. Yes, Revlimid was one of those new, preferred options. Yes, Mayo Clinic was one of the best, if not the best myeloma treatment facilities in the United States! And, yes, the IMF could and would help me battle my insurance company for the right to start using Revlimid as a first course of therapy. Did I know there would be a Patient and Family Seminar in St. Paul in two weeks? I could meet other patients and hear a number of prominent speakers from around the country discuss the latest treatment options.

I learned later the compassionate, knowledgeable voice on the other end of the line was IMF Outreach Director Kelly Cox. I was grateful for our conversation on that down, dark Friday evening. The IMF is a well run organization, and an invaluable resource for any myeloma patients and their families.

The Multiple Myeloma Research Foundation and the Leukemia and Lymphoma Society are also excellent sources of information and support. You can contact the IMF, MMRF and/or the LLS online at www.MultipleMyelomaBlog.com.

Demon Dex

Dexamethasone is the generic name for Decadron, a powerful corticosteroid. The good news is that it is inexpensive. Less than forty dollars for a month's supply. And it works! Dexamethasone can be used to fight myeloma by itself, or in combination with other drugs.

Dex, as it is often called, is much stronger than another commonly used oral steroid, prednisone, The bad news is that dexamethasone comes complete with a long laundry list of possible side effects. A very long list! Cardiac arrest, arrhythmias, cardiac enlargement, congestive heart failure, blood clots, impaired wound healing, hair loss, fluid retention and weight gain, weight loss, abdominal distention, loss of muscle mass, abnormal fat deposits, decreased resistance to infection and osteoporosis just to name a few!

I wasn't thinking about any of this when Dr. Wang prescribed dex for me that day in early April. Four little green tablets, four mg each, taken daily as an anti-inflammatory. I would later learn through reading, seminar presentations and personal experience that dexamethasone can be a very dangerous drug when used over an extended period of time. And I had been using it non-stop for over two months.

I'm not sure why I never connected my early morning insomnia with my dex use. Or the fact that I had lost so much muscle mass and weight during the first month of my treatment. Even if I had inquired about the side effects, it probably wouldn't have made any difference. The dex was working, helping to reduce inflammation in my bones and back and reducing the pain. For better or worse, doctors address and treat the most serious issues first, and worry about negative side effects or lesser complications later.

However, at some point I should have had my dose or frequency adjusted. My extreme and rapid weight loss should have been addressed. But by whom? Dr. Wang? Dr. Zeldenrust? Dr. Smith? In the doctors' defense, things like this can fall between the cracks. (I was so thin, I could have fallen between the cracks!) I had cancer. Cancer patients are expected to lose a lot of weight, right?

While attending the IMF Patient and Caregiver Seminar in St. Paul in June, I overheard a number of conversations among patients and medical staff discussing dexamethasone. I didn't pay much attention. I was uncomfortable and in some pain. But I was alive! I was able to concentrate throughout most of the seven hour presentation, eat lunch with other patients and their families and participate in the small group sessions. Who cared about some inconvenient side effects?

But by early afternoon I was getting a clearer picture about just how insidious dexamethasone could be! One of the earlier speakers spent ten minutes discussing ways to minimize dex's side effects. Later that morning, another speaker proposed possible alternatives to dex and rejoiced when revealing a new "low dose dex" therapy soon to become the standard of care when combined with thalidomide or Revlimid.

Newly completed clinical studies found less was more when using steroids as an adjunct treatment for myeloma—that it actually improved patient survival rates to take less dex. With this proclamation, a large number of attendees began clapping and cheering! I felt the energy level of the room rise noticeably to the point where our speaker and Kelly Cox from the IMF needed to ask everyone to settle down.

Are you kidding me? What were these people talking about? I thought dex was great! It was helping my pain and shrinking my tumors. And besides, the energy boost was amazing! But after another speaker referred to the drug as "Demon Dex," and another "Devil Dex," they began to get my attention.

Until 2006, the standard dosing for dexamethasone had generally been forty mg a day for the first three or four days of a patient's treatment week along with thalidomide or Revlimid. That's three weeks on, followed by one week's rest.

Now I understood. These patients were being forced to endure between one hundred-twenty and one hundred-sixteen mg of dex each week. That's a lot of dexamethasone! No wonder these people were having trouble sleeping for the first part of the week, then crashing at the end. Those poor patients! Then I did more math. I was taking sixteen mg daily. That totaled one hundred-twelve mg each and every week, and I wasn't taking a week to rest.

Looking back, we were all taking too much. Standard dosing now calls for forty mg of dexamethasone at the start of each treatment week. Pulsing the dose in this way tends to isolate most of the negative side effects to two or three days a week, three weeks a month.

The side effects can be annoying. While you are losing muscle mass, you begin to retain water and develop extra belly fat. Not what you want to experience when you are an aging fifty-one year old forced to stop exercising! And did I mention the hair loss, extreme mood swings and feelings of anger and rage? Such adverse reactions are rather inconvenient, especially for the significant other in your life! But there can also be dangerous, even life threatening side effects. More about these later.

I learned an important lesson that day. Networking is important! Talk with other patients. Read as much as you can about myeloma. Find a support group and learn about what works, and doesn't work, for other patients. Prior to attending that seminar, I had no idea dexamethasone was so dangerous. I hadn't thought about treatment options. I blindly followed the advice from my doctors. I'm not even sure that Dr. Anderson would have reduced my dose immediately if I hadn't insisted after sharing what I learned.

After the seminar, Dr. Anderson adjusted my dosing. But it took over a month to wean myself off the steroid completely. I literally had become addicted to dex! Several times after I tried cutting my daily dose by as little as one of the four tablets, I experienced severe cramping in my hands and feet, chills and tremors. I learned I could cut one-half tablet each day and reduce, but not eliminate, these withdrawal symptoms. After six weeks, I was finally able to stop taking dex altogether, just in time to resume taking it again in large, weekly forty mg pulsing doses along with my oral chemotherapy drug, Revlimid.

My Insurance Company Blinks!

I had several concerns about my insurance company's reluctance to fund my Revlimid chemotherapy. The obvious one was the cost. If I couldn't get Blue Cross/Blue Shield to change their mind about paying for Revlimid I had two options. The first was to substitute the more traditional and much harsher thalidomide which, in combination with dexamethasone should be nearly as effective. But I had been warned so many times about the side effects of thalidomide, it didn't seem like a good option.

The second option was to pay for the Revlimid myself. Pattie and I had enough savings to cover the cost of three months at sixty-eight hundred dollars each month. After I told my father about the situation, my supportive parents even offered to pay for the medication. But what about after my transplant? What if the insurance company still refused to pay for the Revlimid then?

That was my biggest concern. Would I need to fight with my insurance company at every turn? The time spent writing letters and on the phone. The anxiety of worrying about our financial stability. The uncertainty of my prognosis and medical future. It was these long term challenges that heightened my levels to what could be damaging levels.

And a more immediate issue was time. I was losing valuable time. I should have already started chemotherapy, and now I had to wait. Worse yet, these delays could affect my transplant schedule at Mayo. If I couldn't complete three months of chemotherapy in time, I would not be able to get started at Mayo in August. Would I lose my place on the transplant waiting list? Would this mean an additional three or four month wait to try again? What would the medical protocol be in the meantime? More expensive drug therapy that insurance wouldn't cover?

Over the next several weeks I found answers to most of my questions. No, I would not have to wait another three or four months to reschedule at Mayo. They would accommodate my drug availability and also help me work with my insurance carrier so we could get started as soon as a decision was made.

While attending the IMF Patient and Family Seminar, I met with a representative from Celgene, the company that manufactures both Revlimid and thalidomide. It turns out Celgene has a non-profit foundation to help patients work with their insurance companies, helping to pay for medications the patients can't afford. I didn't qualify for any long term aid from their foundation, but the company did generously offer to pay for my first month's supply of Revlimid while we got things sorted out! Everyone was optimistic that Blue Cross/ Blue Shield would give in and pay for my medication. We would keep trying.

With backup from Mayo, Dr. Anderson submitted a second insurance reimbursement request for Revlimid. Again, the Medical Management Review Board turned us down! It had now been nearly three weeks since I was scheduled to start my chemotherapy. Normally, someone isn't in a hurry to start chemo, but this delay felt tragic. I needed to get started. I needed to start my battle against cancer NOW!

The next afternoon, after reading Blue Cross/Blue Shield's second rejection letter, I noticed something. The Medical Management Department had again stressed our request did not meet their clinical criteria for use of this drug. It seems the FDA only approved its use after another course of treatment had failed. The IMF, Mayo Clinic and Celgene were all fighting to get Revlimid accepted as a first line treatment for multiple myeloma. But in the meantime, I needed to start treatment yesterday! Why hadn't I thought of this before? I had already received treatment using radiation and dexamethasone. Could something this simple be the answer we were looking for? Had I discovered a loophole that would allow me to press the insurance company to cooperate?

I called Dody at the oncology center in Osceola and asked her to work with Dr. Anderson on another appeal letter based on the new argument- not to expect a change in policy or for the Medical Management Department to make an exception in my case, but only to follow their own specific rules and guidelines.

It worked! My insurance company blinked! Within two weeks, Blue Cross/Blue Shield of Wisconsin had agreed to pay for Revlimid as a second line, ordinary and customary treatment for multiple myeloma. In the meantime, my first prescription for twenty-one, twenty-five mg Revlimid capsules arrived by next day air, paid for by Celgene's Patient Support Solutions Drug Assistance Foundation.

Author's Note: It is already 2012. YES! I'm still alive, almost five years after my diagnosis. And Revlimid is still not approved by the FDA for use in newly diagnosed patients. Fortunately, most insurance companies now approve payment for Revlimid without a fight. But there are several new drugs on the horizon which may not be covered at first. Not to worry! Get your doctor to help you fight any insurance denials you may experience. You can read more about this in the *Insurance* chapter near the end of the book.

A Major Setback

Remember several chapters ago when I wrote we would revisit some of the potentially dangerous side effects one might experience while using a drug like dexamethasone? One of the most serious of these is the possibility of developing blood clots in your legs or, worse yet, your lungs.

Called pulmonary embolus, such clots in your lungs can be life threatening. The risks are heightened when dex is combined with other drugs like Revlimid.

Difficult to treat, these clots can make it hard to breathe and cause a dangerously elevated heart rate. And there is always the risk a part of a clot might move to your heart or brain and kill you! Sound like I know what I'm talking about? I didn't until July of 2007.

Things had been looking up. I won my fight against Blue Cross/Blue Shield so I could start chemotherapy. I began to regain weight as soon as I cut my daily dose of dex and began walking regularly. My mind was clear. I was working, at least part time. Even better, my first month of Revlimid had produced few side effects. Life was good! I had ten weeks to increase my strength and regain some semblance of normalcy before leaving for Rochester to undergo the dreaded stem cell transplant.

But one Saturday, I woke up short of breath with an elevated pulse rate. My normal resting heart rate should be between fifty-five and sixty beats per minute. Now, even at rest, I could not bring my heart rate down below one hundred. I reluctantly allowed Pattie to drive me to the emergency room in Osceola, where I met with a very pleasant but misguided part-time physician who, after ordering a chest x-ray and noticing what might be fluid around my heart, prescribed a diuretic called Furosemide and sent me home.

The previous week I had almost passed out and needed oxygen after the oncology nurses had started an IV for my monthly three hour infusion of Aredia, the bone strengthening biophosphonate I described several chapters back. After Dody and Cathleen fit me with an oxygen mask and cranked up the O2, I was able to continue with my treatment. But not before I was forced to endure some good natured ribbing from them (and my wife) about fainting at the sight of blood!

In spite of the fact I was taking a blood thinner, needed oxygen during my IV, and had an elevated heart-rate, the water retention explanation made sense to me. I had been retaining a lot of water since taking Revlimid. Even before that, my legs had begun to swell, especially my right leg. Everyone said this was to be expected, considering my relative inactivity and the dex. The theory was the water retention was forcing my heart to beat more quickly and elevating my blood pressure, which then caused my shortness of breath.

The most dangerous side effect associated with Revlimid and dexamethasone are blood clots. As a preventative measure, patients are prescribed daily doses of aspirin or a prescription blood thinner like warfarin. I had been taking one eighty-one mg daily dose of aspirin as prescribed by Dr. Anderson for just this reason.

The water retention theory seemed plausible, but I'm not a physician. Between passing out while receiving a simple IV, along with my elevated heart rate and blood pressure, as well as my difficulty breathing, don't you think someone should have suspected I had a blood clot or clots in my legs and lungs?

Monday after the emergency room visit, I saw Dr. Smith for a follow-up. My resting heart rate was still over one hundred beats per minute. There was no improvement by Friday, so I returned to Osceola Medical Center for some additional tests which were inconclusive.

I was unprepared for what followed. Since new chest x-rays didn't help identify the cause of my symptoms, Dr. Smith insisted I be admitted for overnight observation. She felt I needed a CT scan and some additional tests. Except the radioactive die used for these tests is contraindicated for patients with multiple myeloma.

Now suspicious and trying to establish I did indeed have blood clots in my lungs, Dr. Smith scheduled an antiquated, rarely used VQ scan of my lungs for the following day.

Because Osceola Medical Center is a relatively small hospital, my VQ scan would have to be administered in a mobile unit that was parked alongside the hospital building on Saturday mornings. Good timing, I guess. In anticipation of my expected diagnosis I was already taking shots of a blood thinning Heparin type drug called Lovenox.

My resting heart rate was now over one hundred-twenty beats per minute. My blood pressure was up and I was running a fever. And did I mention I still couldn't breathe?

How did I ever find myself in a situation like this? Here I was at age fifty-one, being wheeled down the hall, oxygen tank in tow, feeling weak and very sick. Two young, male med techs used the electronic lift on the back of the truck to get me to the CT machine inside. As an alternative to drinking several liters of chalky fluid or being given a radioactive IV, this throwback VQ test requires you to breathe a medical mist into your lungs for about five minutes before beginning the test. Does anyone see a problem with this? Who would design a test for someone with lung damage that requires deep breathing and holding your breath?

Worse yet, my young assistants did not clearly explain to me how such a test works. I felt panicked and claustrophobic trying to breathe into that mask. For those of you who haven't experienced it, there is nothing more frightening than gasping for air and not being able to breathe! I would start to cough with every other deep breath I was unable to take. The thought of continuing this process throughout an hour long test was unimaginable! "I can't do this, I can't do this anymore!" I gasped as I ripped the VQ mouthpiece from my face and grabbed my oxygen mask to replace it so that I could breathe!

For some reason, the now befuddled med techs thought I meant I could no longer breathe into the mouthpiece at all. What they hadn't explained (and what I didn't know to ask) was I wouldn't be using the mouthpiece once I was pushed into the CT machine and undergoing the actual scan. I could have kept trying had I known that the situation was only temporary.

As things turned out, the scan took an hour and forty minutes because the lack of marker mist in my lungs was not dense enough to allow the machine to do its job. Every breath was a challenge as I lay there sick, in pain, sweating from every pore, barely able to breathe.

That experience helped me empathize with older or chronically ill patients. That day was a real eye opener for me! Being so sick I couldn't even hope to walk to the mailbox. Hooked up to an oxygen tank, unable to breathe deeply into a mouthpiece filled with medicated steam. I now understood what millions of Americans experience every day. How it feels to be old, to be chronically ill, to seem less significant than a normal, healthy human being.

The sketchy test results revealed I did indeed have what looked to be several clots in my lungs. Dr. Smith immediately prescribed an oral blood thinner, warfarin, in addition to the Lovenox shots to dissolve the clots. But things got worse before they began to get better. My temperature spiked, my heart rate continued to race and I felt like crap! Besides the pulmonary embolus, it now become clear to Dr. Smith I was also suffering from bacterial pneumonia. Bring on the IV antibiotics!

It took two days for things to settle down. I still wasn't feeling well. Frustrated, sick and irritable, I had a very bad day Tuesday. Why wasn't I improving? My feelings of frustration only reinforced the uncertainty I had about the future of my health. Medications and treatments were supposed to work. It had always been so! Why was it different for me now? I was losing valuable time! I was supposed to be getting stronger, preparing my body for my upcoming bone marrow transplant in August. I should be walking, lifting weights, eating natural, nutritious foods. Gaining more weight.

My core belief system in medicine and science was shaken. I was beginning to panic. I was gaunt, slumped over. Walking slowly, carefully. I needed an oxygen tank just to shuffle down the hospital halls! And it wasn't getting any better.

My Quick Recovery

You have probably gathered by now that I am not a patient person. Or a good patient, for that matter! The very first goal I set for myself after I was diagnosed with cancer was to be a good patient. I believe how one handles adversity is how one's worth should be measured. It's that athlete's and coach's mentality. As I sat and listened to my chiropractor, Dr. Truhlsen, first tell me I had bone cancer, I was already thinking how I should act and react. Not how I should feel. How I would want or expect to be treated if I were a nurse, doctor or caregiver. To be empathetic. To realize how difficult it must be to care for sick and dying patients. How hard it must be for my chiropractor, who isn't used to handling this type of situation, to look me in the eye and tell me he believed that I was dying!

After four days in the hospital, I was breaking my own rule to be a kind and considerate patient. I was short with my nurse, Dr. Smith and Pattie. My fever was up, I was tired and irritable. "All we can do is wait and give the blood thinners and antibiotics a chance to do their jobs," Dr. Smith repeated. She had stopped by twice a day, and this had become her mantra. "Isn't there anything else we can try?" I would plead. "Pat, I'm sorry. But you have to give it time. This is a serious situation and we need to monitor you closely." It's not like I was going anywhere. I had needed oxygen continually since I had arrived.

Fortunately, the next day was better! My blood had thinned and my INR was now elevated enough so I no longer needed two daily shots of Lovenox. I began to improve by the hour. I learned later I was allergic to Lovenox! Those allergic reactions contributed to my unusually high fever. By a wonderful coincidence, the same time I stopped receiving the Lovenox injections, the IV antibiotics kicked in and BAM! I felt much, much better Wednesday.

After a final infusion of antibiotics Thursday morning, I was able to return home, oxygen tank in tow. I was weak and shaken, sick from my clots, pneumonia and chemo, but none of that mattered. I was home, laying in my own bed! I would soon be back on track. Tomorrow would be better. I would live to fight another day!

Doctors Are People Too!

I would like to pause here for a moment and reflect back on my hospital stay. A number of mistakes were made. A number of things went wrong. Now I am not being critical of Dr Smith. This is really about communication. Had Dr. Anderson known about my situation earlier, he may have picked up the telltale signs of a clot.

Who was responsible to get this information to Dr. Anderson? If you think about it, I was! Had I been better informed and paid attention to the warnings and literature included with my medications, maybe I would have known enough to express my concerns to Dr. Smith or directly to Dr. Anderson. We hear and read so many disclaimers about medications we become numb to the fine print. Big mistake!

Ultimately I believe we, as patients, are responsible for their own medical care.

Doctors are people too! They make mistakes, get distracted, have bad days or don't know all the facts concerning your case. Often the only constant while a patient is being shuffled from doctor to doctor and department to department is YOU!

Recently my father started taking medication for an irregular heartbeat. One of the possible side effects of this particular medication, Cordarone, is the thickening of lung tissue over time. Noticing this was a common side effect, my father systematically collected copies of his radiology reports and x-rays. After several years he noticed subtle shadows on his films that weren't there before. He also found mention of this buried deep in his most recent radiology report. After bringing these findings to the attention of his cardiologist, he was immediately prescribed a substitute medication. He now gets a chest x-ray every six months and the progression of the infiltrate, as it is called, has halted.

Now I am not suggesting we all need to be radiologists or M.D.'s. But think about it. After the initial shock of your diagnosis wears off and your emotional and medical situation stabilizes, who can be more of an expert on your medical condition than you? If you listen to each nurse and physician carefully, you can learn a lot. Talk with your med techs about why you are taking a test and what it means. Ask your nurses what they would do if they were you and what they think. Make sure each doctor gets a full picture of your medical condition by hand delivering reports and taking notes. Ask lots of questions. Whenever possible, bring a friend, family member or caregiver along with you to your appointment to take notes and listen with a second set of ears. Better yet, have the same person serve that function as often as possible. Now you have someone else close to the situation who might catch what you or your medical team misses!

What about my allergic reaction to Lovenox? It was the Lovenox injections causing my fever, aches and chills. Chalk that up to bad luck. No one could have known about that. Allergic reactions to this injectable blood thinner are very rare. I later connected my symptoms to Lovenox after returning from treatment at Mayo Clinic months later.

Of course, if you try to monitor and understand every potential side effect of your medication, even something as common as aspirin, you can drive yourself crazy with worry! As with all things in life, balance is the key. If I knew exactly how to help you find that balance, I would certainly share that wisdom with you—from my new yacht in the Caribbean!

Stem Cell Transplant?

When I was diagnosed with multiple myeloma in April 2007, it was assumed I would soon be receiving a stem cell transplant. I had much to learn about the process.

There are two basic types of transplants: autologous and allogeneic. Autologous is the most common type for lymphatic and bone marrow cancers. An autologous transplant uses a patient's own bone marrow stem cells, which are harvested prior to the procedure.

In an allogeneic transplant, healthy stem cells are taken from a parent, other family member or unrelated matching donor with similar blood and marrow types. Stem cells can also sometimes be collected from an umbilical cord that was frozen and stored at birth.

As with any transplant that uses donor tissue, anti-rejection drugs are necessary to help the recipient's body fight off graft-versus-host disease. This is a negative reaction of white blood cells in transplanted tissue against the tissues of the recipient, or host.

In theory, an allogeneic transplant gives a multiple myeloma patient his or her best chance of achieving long term remission. Yet this procedure is rarely used, except as a last resort in myeloma patients, for several reasons. First, the risk of complications during and immediately after the procedure is high. Second, surviving patients may need to take anti-rejection drugs for the remainder of their lives. These drugs often carry their own risks and side effects. Third, the possibility of serious graft-versus-host disease can make post transplant recuperation difficult. Finally, it is often very challenging to find a compatible donor.

For most myeloma patients, an allogeneic transplant is not a good option. A friend of mine named Steve from Roseville, Minnesota, needed an allogeneic transplant. His last stand, new age combination chemotherapy regimen of Revlimid, Velcade and dexamethasone had started to slip, meaning his myeloma was becoming more active and dangerous. Steve had already survived one stem cell transplant. But he didn't have enough stored cells to complete transplant number two.

Steve has three brothers, but no one in his family was an acceptable match. His oncologist hoped to find an unrelated donor.

Several weeks after hearing about his situation, I ran into Steve at a multiple myeloma seminar, sponsored by the International Myeloma Foundation in St Louis Park, Minnesota. Steve felt good. Things were going OK. His numbers, while slipping, were not so bad. Hopefully a donor could be found during the next few months.

A Myeloma and transplant specialist, Dr. Angela Dispenzieri from the Mayo Clinic, was the morning speaker at the seminar. Steve was sitting about twenty seats away from me in the front row. Aware of his situation, I looked over toward him as Dr. Dispenzieri began to discuss allogeneic trasplants as part of her presentation. She stated an allogeneic transplant offered the greatest hope of true remission. Steve was leaning forward, expressionless, listening carefully. But as Dr. Dispenzieri went on to cover the procedure's risks, I could see the color drain from Steve's face. His jaw dropped and he slumped back in his chair as the doctor mentioned that until recently, thirty percent of allogeneic transplant patients don't survive the procedure!

I had never known the survival rate had been so low. Obviously, neither did Steve! Dr Dispenzieri later quoted a current rate of fifteen percent, which was closer to what I understood the percentage to be.

Using a more positive spin, Dr. Dispenzieri went on to emphasize this means a patient has an eighty-five percent chance of surviving. Still, considering the survival rate for patients undergoing an autologous transplant was over ninety-nine percent, this was a pretty sobering number for Steve to hear!

We joked a bit about it at lunch after the presentation. Steve seemed fine with everything. But I could tell his confidence had been shaken. Reality can really bite!

My editor, Julie, made a simple notation at this point on my manuscript: "What happened to Steve?"

Steve and I last spoke in late October, 2008. He was hanging in there, but his physicians all still agreed, despite the risks, that his best option was to undergo an allogeneic transplant. Steve was still waiting for a compatible donor. If such a donor could not be found in time, doctors would try a transplant using cells taken from donated umbilical cord blood.

Other, less common and more controversial transplant options than allogeneic transplants are mini-allogeneic transplants, stem cell transplants using cells from umbilical cords and tandem autologous transplants.

Mini-allogeneic transplants are a less aggressive, less dangerous form of allogeneic stem cell transplant. Transplants using donor umbilical cord cells are safer still. Both of these options are less common and more experimental than autologous or allogeneic transplants.

Tandem autologous transplants were pioneered at the Myeloma Institute in Arkansas. According to the Multiple Myeloma Research Foundation, tandem transplants are planned, back to back autologous stem cell transplants performed within six months of each other. Although back to back transplants are hard for a patient to tolerate, some data supports their use as a way to help patients achieve a longer lasting complete response. The question is, does the risk of complications and discomfort of the patient justify the results?

As the efficacy of new myeloma chemotherapy drugs has improved, tandem transplants have lost favor with the majority of myeloma treatment centers and are not considered a standard of care.

Still, an autologous transplant is sometimes repeated when the first transplant doesn't work well. For this reason, oncologists often recommend collecting enough stem cells during a patient's harvest for more than one transplant.

Autologous transplants can be relatively safe. But they are, by nature, a flawed procedure. Think about it. The surgeon removes a cancer patient's own stem cells to reintroduce later after the remaining bone marrow is destroyed. This avoids anti-rejection issues that make an allogeneic transplant so dangerous. But it also means no matter how effective a patient's chemotherapy regimen was prior to the transplant, the re-introduced stem cells were still exposed to cancer.

But according to Dr Dispenzieri, there are other more likely reasons that autologous transplants eventually fail. She feels there is something in a patient's physiological makeup that allows the cancer to return.

The most likely cause of relapse may be that a number of hidden Myeloma cells in a patient's body that is not destroyed during pre-transplant chemotherapy. This is probably why many myeloma patients who undergo an allogeneic transplant also eventually relapse. So even if a patient is fortunate enough to receive an infusion of cancer free stem cells, the basic DNA of the plasma cells that allows the cancer to get started in the first place hasn't changed. Unfortunately as described above, the cancer is almost surely destined to return.

The terms "bone marrow transplant" and "stem cell transplant" are often incorrectly used interchangeably. In the 1980's and early 1990's, autologous and allogeneic transplants were performed surgically by extracting stem cells from the bone marrow using needles. Now it is far more common to collect stem cells from a patient's circulating blood by a process called apheresis. A transplant using stem cells collected this way is called a stem cell transplant. The term blood and marrow transplant (BMT) covers both procedures.

Much safer than a decade ago, stem cell transplants are still a dangerous and invasive procedure. A 99% survival rate is fine, unless you are one of the 1%! Not to mention the discomfort of having your bone marrow chemically destroyed and any non-lethal complications or side effects. Mayo Clinic prefers to try and work with recipients as out-patients. But if anything goes wrong, a patient is immediately hospitalized. Other highly rated transplant centers like the University of Minnesota Hospital or Duke Medical Center in North Carolina prefer to hospitalize patients for the first two or three weeks as they slowly transition to out-patient status.

I was given a preliminary transplant schedule recommending that I plan to stay in Rochester for up to ten weeks as an out-patient. Ten weeks! That is a lot of time to spend away from home, not working. Just as inconvenient is the following two to three months spent recuperating with low energy levels and various uncomfortable side effects to work through.

You don't need a medical degree to understand undergoing a stem cell transplant is no fun!

Yet there are some positives. I know transplant recipients who have lived five, six, even seven years cancer free. That means years of living a normal life, sometimes without drugs! Another plus is often, drug therapies that lose their effectiveness prior to transplantation begin to work again. And although this is a very expensive undertaking (stem cell transplants can cost up to one hundred-fifty thousand dollars!) transplantation is considered the standard of care in most myeloma cases for patients under seventy five-years of age. That means insurance companies are likely to pay for most, if not all, of the bills associated with the transplant process. This can be an advantage since many insurance companies are reluctant to pay for newer chemotherapy drugs that they consider experimental.

The bottom line in 2007—a stem cell transplant remained the standard of care for most myeloma patients. I didn't realize it at the time of my diagnosis, but this was beginning to change.

The book, *Everyone's Guide to Cancer Therapy,* notes, "Ninety percent of all drug cures occur in just over ten percent of cancer types." Lucky me! Multiple myeloma is near the top of the list of cancers that respond well to chemotherapy intervention.

New drugs like Revlimid and Velcade are revolutionizing the treatment of multiple myeloma. Combination therapies using these and other drugs are giving oncologists a wide variety of weapons to slow the progress of the cancer. Not cure it, mind you. But slow it down enough to help improve a patient's quality of life.

When I met with Dr. Zeldenrust in May of 2007, there was still no clinical evidence any of these therapies extended a patient's life. This seemed counterintuitive to me! "So Dr. Zeldenrust, what happens if my Revlimid and dexamethasone therapy continues to work for years?" "You will live an average of forty-three months," he replied stoically. "So if I then undergo a successful stem cell transplant that works for years?" "Dr. Zeldenrust cut me off. "You will probably live about forty-three months." He continued, "Remember that forty-three months is an average. You may very well live longer. But there is no statistical evidence that the type or timing of the treatment that you undergo will extend your life. It is more a quality of life issue." He went on to explain a stem cell transplant allows a patient to live a normal life without drugs for years following the procedure. It doesn't matter if you get the transplant first and try all the available chemotherapy drugs second. Or if you use the drug combinations first and then try a transplant in the end. There is no statistical difference. Dr. Zeldenrust concluded by using this analogy. "Think about it like you are going to pull off a band-aid. You can slowly pull the band-aid back or you can rip it off. Either way, it is going to hurt! Some people like to take it slow and try the drugs first. These drugs are very expensive and often cause a number of side effects. But eventually they will need to use the transplant option." He continued. "Others decide to get the transplant right away before their body is weakened by extended chemotherapy. There is no right or wrong way to do this. The only question is when!"

Once again, Dr. Zeldenrust had been blunt and direct. The facts were the facts. Someday I would need a transplant.

Author Note: More good news here! OK. We have established it is difficult to assign median life expectancy numbers to newly diagnosed myeloma patients these days. But most cancer patients want–no need, and sometimes even demand–a prognosis.

So what are oncologists at regional cancer centers telling their newly diagnosed patients now in 2012? Lacking any real consensus among specialists, honest myeloma docs across the country are most likely looking their patients in the eyes and saying "We just don't know." But realizing "We just don't know." is an unacceptable answer for nearly any cancer patient, most specialists would share life expectancy estimates of anywhere between seven and ten years. That's more than double the length of my prognosis in 2007!

What about the inevitability of needing a stem cell transplant? Want to hear more good news? Although somewhat controversial, a growing number of myeloma experts have concluded stem cell transplants are becoming just one of a growing number of treatment options. More and more patients are choosing to delay their transplant in the hope they may never need to undergo the procedure. I discuss the pros and cons of transplantation later in the chapter, Dealing with Treatment Options.

But What About Velcade?

Revlimid is one of a handful of new multiple myeloma chemotherapy drugs known as novel therapy agents–thalidomide, or Thalomid, is another. Both Revlimid and Thalomid are administered orally. A third novel therapy agent, Velcade, is delivered through an IV-push.

Approved for use against multiple myeloma in 2003, Velcade, the trade name for bortezomid, is part of a new class of cancer drugs called proteasome inhibitors. Like Revlimid, Velcade was originally only approved for use in previously treated multiple myeloma patients. That all changed in June of 2008 when Velcade was also approved by the FDA for use in newly diagnosed patients.

Velcade has been around long enough to develop an impressive track record of improvement in a majority of myeloma patients that try the drug. So why did Dr. Zeldenrust start me on Revlimid instead of Velcade?

First, since he knew I lived over two hours away from the Mayo Clinic in Rochester, Dr. Zeldenrust felt it would be more convenient for me to take Revlimid capsules, as opposed to traveling for an IV treatment eight or more times each month. Second, Revlimid tends to work more quickly than Velcade. Since I was originally scheduled to undergo a stem cell transplant three or four months after our initial consultation, Revlimid was a solid choice.

But it wasn't the only approved option. Dr. Zeldenrust could have chosen to start me on Thalomid or Velcade instead. Like Revlimid, in most cases the steroid, dexamethasone, would also be used along with the primary chemotherapy drug. And although combination therapies were not commonly used at the time of my diagnosis in April of 2007, a number of highly rated cancer centers like the University of Arkansas Multiple Myeloma Research Center in Little Rock, Dana Farber in Boston, Cedars Sinai in Los Angeles and Moffitt Cancer Center in Tampa are now all starting to use multiple combinations of novel therapies pre-transplant.

Multiple combinations of Thalomid/Velcade/dex, or Revlimid/Velcade/dex are becoming more and more common. An additional drug, Doxil, is sometimes added to the mix as well. Clinical trials have proven Velcade works best when combined with other anti-myeloma drugs.

I now know there are several advantages to starting newly diagnosed patients on Velcade. Recent studies have found using Revlimid pre-transplant can make the collection of a patient's stem cells more difficult. Using Velcade rarely affects a patient's ability to harvest stem cells.

In addition, there are possible insurance and financial considerations. Since Velcade is administered through an IV, Medicare Part B and most Insurance companies cover the cost of Velcade. Thalomid and Revlimid are oral medications and are often only covered under a prescription drug plan. Even though taking a capsule orally may be a bit more convenient, the high cost of these oral therapies can make Velcade a more affordable choice.

Velcade is manufactured by Millennium Pharmaceuticals, which is now owned by Takeda Oncology Company of Japan. I recently visited Millennium's facilities on the campus of MIT in Cambridge, Massachusetts. The staff and facilities are both first-rate. But what impressed me most was a briefing about a number of promising new myeloma fighting drugs that Millennium is already testing in advanced clinical trials. Multiple myeloma patients should be excited and hopeful–more help is on the way!

Dealing with Treatment Options

Dealing with treatment options is a challenge most cancer patients face. At first you tend to accept the recommendations of your doctors without question. Often the decisions are simple and direct. There is a consensus between treating physicians and nurses on the best way to proceed. This seemed to be the case here.

There is a certain comfort in being led. In being told what to do. After all, the doctors are the experts! I was physically and emotionally weak. If my oncologist says I should get a transplant, that is what I would do!

Four days after I met with Dr. Zeldenrust in Rochester, I received my transplant itinerary in the mail. It was quite impressive! Nine pages of scheduled meetings, tests and procedures. Three days of preliminary testing to make sure

I was healthy enough to undergo a transplant. Four days for growth factor injections that would force my marrow to begin producing extra stem cells that could then be harvested by running my blood through an aphaeresis machine for an additional three to six days. Once the desired number of cells were harvested, my bone marrow would be destroyed using a strong chemotherapy agent. A day or two later, my own stem cells would be infused back into my body in the hope they would graft and begin to produce new, cancer free bone marrow. Six to eight weeks after that I would be headed home, tired but hopefully cancer free for years to come.

There it was, all structured and organized. My itinerary. "You're young!" the doctors and nurses would say. "You're so young and strong! You will be just fine." I heard again and again. It seems that most patients don't undergo a transplant until they are in their sixties or sometimes, early to mid-seventies. To my new medical team, I was young and strong. But I sure didn't feel that way!

I watched a DVD produced by the Mayo Clinic about BMT's. The key, according to the DVD, was your caregiver. He or she would need to be there to help you get to appointments, take your medications as prescribed and later help feed you and keep you moving on days when you just didn't want to move.

I had not seen my parents since my diagnosis and treatment in April. Their home in Rockford, Illinois, was about a five hour drive away. Everyone had agreed it would be best if my parents didn't visit until things were more stable, and I wasn't so sick. The counseling staff I met with in May recommended caregivers and family also view the DVD so they could get an overview of the challenges ahead.

My parents had been so worried about me they were more than happy to make the five hour drive north to visit. We hugged, toured the area (which is beautiful, by the way) and ate dinner at a magnificent area restaurant, Paradise Landing, on an outdoor terrace overlooking Balsam Lake. We then returned home to watch the DVD together.

It was a difficult forty minutes. The DVD itself was harmless enough. It gave a sugar coated rundown of the transplant process, and what patient and family would most likely be forced to bear. My father, Ted, sat silently throughout. My mother, Jean, commented positively in her usual animated and supportive fashion a number of times during the presentation. Pattie fidgeted nervously and worked cleaning the kitchen, watching for my reaction to the DVD. All I could focus on was the upcoming pain, discomfort and recovery time away from home and work.

First, they shoot you full of growth hormone to get your stem cell production to explode. Next they kill all of your bone marrow. Then your stem cells are reintroduced, along with a preservative chemical that makes you sick and jaundiced. Hopefully the new cells begin to grow, and after suffering hair loss, mouth and throat sores, extreme fatigue and one or more bouts with viral shingles, you get to go home after about ten weeks. A friend who completed his transplant the year before had a relatively easy experience, but still needed several additional months of rest at home before he could work more than four or five hours a day. Sounded like a vacation to me!

What about Pattie? She would need to care for me, try to keep our real estate practice on life support, take care of our rescued dogs and cats, and continue to help her mother who was living nearby in assisted living. I was overwhelmed with grief, frustration and emotion. Why was this happening to me? I DON'T WANT TO DO THIS!

I tried not to let my fear and frustration show. I'm not sure I did a very good job.

My parents left the following day after taking us out to a big breakfast. I was still fourteen pounds below my normal, healthy weight. It seemed clear I would need all the strength I could muster to withstand my chemotherapy regimen and get ready for my transplant, which would now have to be rescheduled for September. Bring out the pancakes! And the butter!

Over the next week or so I overcame my initial aversion to my inevitable transplant and embraced the challenge! It was as if someone had flipped a switch. I guess I just needed to grieve and allow myself to get angry. Overnight I started to look at my impending transplant in a more positive light. It was time to stop feeling sorry for myself and get on with the rest of my life!

Pattie and I scheduled another trip to Rochester to explore our housing options while I would be receiving outpatient care. Many patients chose to stay at the Transplant House, a nondenominational, independently operated facility with patient and guest rooms, a nice kitchen, family lounge and old style covered front porch about three blocks from Mayo Clinic. Priced less than thirty dollars per night, this home-style boarding facility was immaculately clean and structured to meet the needs of recovering transplant patients. We soon discovered this was not the best option for us. Televisions and computers were not allowed in patients' rooms. Caregivers were required to stay and sleep with the patient at all times. Meals were prepared by the patient or caregiver in a communal kitchen. Strict rules were in place to protect the health of the residents. There was a TV lounge and computer room. The philosophy here was to give patients and their families a chance to meet and share with others in a similar position. Sort of like a live-in support group. This communal set-up was intentionally designed to encourage patients to get out of their room to move and socialize. It was truly a special place.

Now I know a number of people who stayed in the Transplant House and loved it. The price was certainly right! But the environment felt too restrictive for us. No TV in the room? That was a deal breaker for both of us right there! We decided instead to lease an extended stay motel suite about seven blocks away from the clinic. Still close enough to walk to Mayo except on my sickest of days, this two room sweet would allow visitors and guests to stay with us while they were visiting. There was a pool for Pattie to use in the main building along with a breakfast buffet each morning. The room featured a small kitchen, convenient parking, high speed Internet and yes, a TV in each room. The cost was more than twice as much as the Transplant House, but convenience and accommodations for family and other visitors justified the price.

Concerned Pattie would be overwhelmed with my care and other obligations, I called my sister Peg, in Texas, and my brother, John, and my other sister, Joan, both from the Chicago area, and asked if they could come and stay with me in three or four day shifts. That would allow Pattie to spend some time at home with the animals and to catch up on work. All generously agreed to help. My college roommate, Tim Hanna, from Appleton, Wisconsin, along with Pattie's sister, Mary, from Florida, also volunteered to help care for me during my stay.

I carefully crafted a rotating schedule based on each caregiver's availability, and mailed copies to all along with information about the area and a list of their responsibilities so they would know what to expect. I joked with Pattie this would be a national team effort! I was touched and energized by the support pledged by friends and family.

Our plan was to have two cars in Rochester. One for Pattie to use commuting the two plus hours back and forth every few days between Rochester and St Croix Falls. The other would be available for my sister, Peg, or brother, John, to use after they flew in to stay. I was so proud of myself as I carefully laid out the specifics of my plan down to the last detail, and included them on my color coded caregivers schedule. For example, Pattie would pick up Peg or John at the airport, stay to help acclimate them to my situation and new surroundings, then drive north to spend three or four days back home.

There was only one important contingency for which I had not planned. What if I didn't need my transplant after all?

Remember this chapter is titled "Dealing with Treatment Options." What I had not foreseen was the possibility it might be better to delay or even cancel my plans for a stem cell transplant.

The summer of 2007 was an exciting time for medical professionals and their patients dealing with multiple myeloma. Both new chemotherapy drugs, Revlimid and Velcade, were beginning to exceed even the most optimistic projections for their effectiveness. These drugs were still being used in clinical trials and had not yet produced any long term data to help guide oncologists as how to best use them. What was the most effective dose? Frequency of application? What were the long term effects on patients bodies using the drugs by themselves or in different combinations? Oncologists only knew both drugs, used alone or in a variety of combinations, were working.

My medical oncologist, Dr. Anderson, had asked me to consider delaying my transplant several times. Why? The Rev/dex combination therapy I had started in May was already working! Some improvement was expected and necessary to help assure a successful transplant. But my improvement had been fast and exceeded all expectations.

How did we know that? Three protein markers are traditionally used to track the progression of multiple myeloma. The most important is a patient's "M-spike." This blood test searches for the presence of any monoclonal protein in the bloodstream. A healthy person with normal levels of serum protein electrophoresis will have an M-spike of zero. When I was first diagnosed, my M-spike was five. That was very high. Dr. Zeldenrust wanted to see my number well below two before I proceeded to transplant.

The other most common tests also measure two different types of protein in the patient's blood. Along with an M-spike, IgG and IgA markers are used to monitor myelom'a activity. Both of these numbers also started out very high, well over three thousand. Normal IgG numbers should be between six hundred and fourteen hundred mg and normal IgA numbers between eighty and three hundred-forty mg.

After less than three months of treatment, my M-spike had dropped all the way down below one, and my other two protein markers were within or below the normal range! My radiation and dexamethasone therapy in April had already improved those numbers. The Rev/dex combination had accelerated my improvement throughout May and June. My hospitalization at the beginning of June may have been a frustrating physical setback, but it did nothing to slow the progress of this new, expensive, wonder drug called Revlimid!

My numbers held and even dropped slightly through July and into August. My monoclonal protein level was now down to point four, which was barely measurable.

And my IgG and IgA numbers remained in or below the normal range.

It seemed like a miracle! True, I often felt flu-like and had to deal with other annoying side effects. But the drugs were working! Or was it the prayers of my family and friends? After all, I was on every church prayer list in the area! And in my parents' church in Rockford. And my brother and sister's churches in Illinois and Texas. I was receiving encouraging phone calls, cards and e-mails from other Realtors, clients and community business owners. I was deeply touched!

Was it the drugs, prayers, nutrition, my strong, positive mental attitude or Pattie's love and support? Yes! Yes to all of the above!

About this time I started attending myeloma support group meetings in Stillwater, Minnesota, about forty minutes from my home. There I learned a number of survivors had opted not to get a transplant. They too had experienced positive results using Revlimid or thalidomide, and had decided to wait.

Surprisingly, I fought the idea of waiting at first. I was so invested in my planning for a transplant I was having trouble letting go. I didn't want to "wimp out" and choose to wait because the procedure was so unpleasant! But what I hadn't stopped to consider was a stem cell transplant is more than unpleasant. It is an aggressive, invasive procedure with serious risks and side effects.

The year before, a friend of mine, Loren Leidl, had himself undergone a stem cell transplant at Mayo Clinic. Loren's experience had been positive. Yes, he was tired for months following his stay in Rochester. But everything had gone according to plan and the results were good.

So you can imagine my surprise when Loren suggested on several occasions I delay my scheduled transplant! "Always use your conservative options first," Loren would say. "My transplant wasn't any big deal, but I know people who have had real problems during and after their transplants."

Loren is a hero of mine. He has been battling multiple myeloma for almost twelve years. That is an eternity in the myeloma survival business! In 2007, only ten percent of myeloma patients survived ten years or more. That number quickly fell to five percent or less after twelve years. Yet here he was, working part-time and spending priceless days with friends and family, acting like he would live forever! Loren tried every available drug and treatment more than once. "Everything that I have tried seems to work for about fourteen months. The only drug that didn't work well for me was Revlimid. I had an allergic skin reaction to the drug that makes it almost impossible for me to use." Loren went on to explain, ironically, his stem cell transplant had only worked for about ten months. Of all the many therapies he tried, the most dangerous and invasive one worked for the shortest period of time. That really got me thinking!

The possibility my transplant wouldn't be effective or last very long had always been one of my concerns. The average transplant only works for about eighteen months. Over the course of the summer, I talked with a number of people who had friends whose transplants didn't last. One unfortunate member of our support group, Sharon Quast, needed to start chemotherapy within three months of her transplant after her procedure failed to eliminate the cancer in her bone marrow. That is a lot of lost time, pain and riskto undergo for a procedure that didn't work!

Of course, I also knew people whose had transplants that had worked for years. Another support group member, Iwona Srienc from Lake Elmo, Minnesota, had an autologous blood and marrow transplant in 1997 that is still working today! But even Iwona told me she would consider waiting if she were me. It is one thing to try an aggressive therapy or surgery when you don't have any other choice like my friend, Steve. But it was becoming clear that I might have other options.

Around this time another close friend of mine, Gene Krushek, called to see how I was holding up. Gene worked for Kodak out of St Paul. I had helped him find some land on a small lake near St. Croix Falls in 2004. We kept in touch and the following year Gene decided to try selling real estate part-time as he transitioned into retirement. I helped him get started with my former company, Century 21 Premier Group. After I switched real estate companies and began working for Mike Muske at ERA, the plan was for Gene to join me in our new St Croix Falls office mid-summer of 2006.

I was shocked when Gene stopped by that June and told me he had been diagnosed with bone cancer the day before, and was informed by his physician he only had three months to live! This was many months before my diagnosis, so I couldn't imagine how it felt to be blindsided by the fact your life could end so abruptly and unexpectedly. My partner, Bruce, and I sat stunned as Gene explained he had an advanced case of prostate cancer that had metastasized to his bone. There was no cure.

That next week, Gene and his wife, Roxy, visited several specialists who confirmed the diagnosis. One suggested that an extreme type of chemotherapy might extend his life by six months or so, if he survived the treatments!

Undeterred, Genevisited a cancer treatment center in Zion, Illinois. He wasn't comfortable with their recommendation, so he continued to do his own research. Gene ended up going to a smaller cancer clinic in the Twin Cities that proposed a far less intense course of treatment using a combination of hormone therapy and nutrition. More than one year later, here was Gene calling to check how I was feeling! He was able to continue working (in part to keep his health insurance!) and using his accumulated vacation time to travel and spend more time with Roxy.

Gene listened carefully as I laid out my treatment options. Gene is a quiet, thoughtful guy, but without hesitation he abruptly said, "Don't get the transplant!" "Pat," he continued, "that sounds like a dangerous procedure. Always go with the safer, more conservative treatment option first."

I was surprised by his assertiveness. This was a major medical decision. If it were me, I might be more careful and measured with my advice. But not Gene! "Look how well the conservative approach has worked for me!" he added. "When in doubt, wait!"

Even before I began my chemotherapy, Pattie had wanted me to delay as well. "Let's wait and see what happens first," she had said. But ultimately the decision was up to me and she was supportive whatever I chose to do. It was time to decide.

The first call I made was to Dr. Zeldenrust. I was following up on a letter I mailed to him the week before, outlining my thoughts and concerns regarding the impending transplant. Wouldn't it be better to wait and save my transplant for when the various drug combinations were no longer working?

In an impressive display of professionalism and concern, Dr. Zeldenrust spent over forty minutes with me on the phone, going over the pros and cons of my transplant's timing. Dr. Zeldenrust conceded the recent success of the new drugs had cast doubt on using a stem cell transplant as the standard of care for myeloma patients under seventy years of age. He shared a story with me in which he described how a promising study of Revlimid had recently failed. Not because things didn't go well, but because the results were too successful! Apparently, this particular study planned to follow the progress of myeloma patients after they took the Revlimid/dex combination for one year. Then those patients were to stop taking the drugs so doctors could better understand how and when the cancer would return. The Rev/dex combination worked so well, most of the patients refused to stop taking the drugs, even if forced to pay for them themselves!

As a result, Dr. Zeldenrust explained we don't know enough about how our bodies react after using Revlimid over a long period of time. Are there any lasting side effects? Would the cancer return shortly after a patient discontinued its use, or would the cancer stay dormant for an extended period of time?

What he could tell me was a majority of patients were OK after eighteen months, matching the success rate of the average autologous transplant! Without evidence to the contrary, a logical person could conclude they would be better off using the very expensive, but equally effective drug, as long as one could afford the cost. "What about the wisdom of selecting the most conservative, least risky treatment available to treat this and any other type of cancer?" I asked. "Always a good idea!" he responded affirmatively.

Dr. Zeldenrust's only caveat was the fact I was doing so well made me a prime candidate for transplant. He insisted that I keep my scheduled appointment at Mayo to have my stem cells harvested for future transplant. But as long as that was done as soon as possible, Dr. Zeldenrust could see no reason why I couldn't, or shouldn't, wait.

Author's Note: I was able to achieve a complete response (CR), or remission after 14 months. I stayed in CR for over two years, using only a low maintenance dose of Revlimid. Unfortunately, my myeloma inevitably became active again late in 2010. After needing radiation to zap a new, large lesion in my right hip, Pattie and I decided that I should undergo a stem cell transplant after all. Four years after my initial diagnosis, I underwent an autologous (using my stem cells) stem cell transplant in the summer of 2011 at Moffitt Cancer Center in Tampa, Florida.

While at Moffitt, I interviewed dozens of other stem cell transplant patients, including several who had experienced an allogeneic transplant, using stem cells from a donor. I share my transplant experience in my second book, *Stem Cell Transplants from a Patient's Perspective*. The 344 page book is packed-full of tips and advice from those who understand the process best; the patients.

Ironically, despite the fact I was a prime candidate, my stem cell transplant did not work. But fortunately, a combination of Revlimid, Velcade and dexamethasone (RVD) has been able to hold my myeloma in check, post transplant.

Las Vegas!

Pick your metaphor. If life gives you lemons, make lemonade! If a door closes, a window opens!

In late August, 2007, I returned to Mayo Clinic for my pre-stem cell harvest testing; three intense days of testing and consultations to ready us for my stem cell harvest, which was now scheduled to begin over Labor Day weekend.

The test results and news were good. Better than good, they were great! My blood work continued to be excellent, with a barely measurable M-spike and low to normal IgG and IgA readings. My bones were beginning to heal. The combination of time and my biophosphonate, Aredia, were having measurable results. Best of all, my bone marrow biopsy (sedated, of course!) showed no detectable cancer cells. None! A normal plasma cell count in a healthy person's bone marrow should be less than 5%. When I was diagnosed, mine was over thirty percent! Now it was down to five percent and the Mayo Clinic pathologists could find no evidence of cancer there.

Great news, right? Not according to my insurance company. I was doing too well, they said, to justify paying for my stem cell harvest! They would not pay to collect and store my stem cells.

This was a problem. I spoke with the patient aid department at Mayo and we determined the average collect and store cost was about thirty thousand dollars. Once again my parents stepped up and, without my asking, offered to pay for the procedure. Still, this seemed very short-sighted on the insurance company's part.

Crazier yet was the next twist. Blue Cross/Blue Shield would pay for the collect and store if I continued on and had my transplant right away! In other words, I was too healthy to collect my stem cells to use later when I needed them. But if I then scheduled and completed my transplant within three months of my collection, Blue Cross/Blue Shield would pay all of the estimated one hundred-fifty thousand dollars to complete the transplant, including one year's follow up care.

Now was the time to collect my cells! I was relatively cancer free, and my stem cells should still be strong and not weakened from months or years of chemotherapy and radiation. But Dr. Anderson and Dr. Zeldenrust both assured me that a few extra months would probably not make any difference, so I decided not to proceed without insurance. I was disillusioned, yet confident that Blue Cross/Blue Shield would eventually change their minds.

Have I mentioned my wife, Pattie, and I are huge University of Wisconsin Badgers fans? We both graduated from the University of Wisconsin and followed the football, basketball and hockey teams religiously. Each of the past three years, we traveled to Florida to watch the UW football team play in a New Year's Day bowl game. This year the team had scheduled a regular season game against the University of Las Vegas on September 9th.

Now, Pattie and I are not your typical Las Vegas type visitors. We don't gamble, drink (much) or like really hot weather. But we traveled there a number of times on business, and loved to watch the crazy people and experience the lights and excitement of the Las Vegas Strip. The last time we were there for a meeting, Pattie and I heard stories about how crazy Badger fans were the year before when they played in Las Vegas. One of our cab drivers noticed my red UW shirt and went on and on about the sea of red (UW's team colors are red and white) he watched as he drove up and down the strip. He also laughed as he told us how many of the casinos ran out of beer that weekend. Badger fans love to party!

Ever since then, Pattie and I had talked about traveling west if the Badgers ever played again in Las Vegas. And there it was on the schedule. September 9th, 2007. Our University of Wisconsin Badgers were going to play the University of Las Vegas Running Rebels. We had planned a trip to the game for over a year. I kidded Pattie I thought she was more disappointed to be missing the game than about the fact I was scheduled to start my transplant that week. She even asked Dr. Zeldenrust to schedule the transplant a week later so we could still go to the game.

Dr. Zeldenrust didn't think that would be a good idea. My position was always not to mess with Mayo! If the Mayo Clinic scheduled me for the first week in September, that's when it would be! My collect and store might be complete in time to leave for the game, but everything would have to go just right. And if we postponed there was no guarantee when we could re-schedule.

But thanks to the insurance company, my collect and store was indefinitely postponed! We got to make lemonade! The door closed, the window opened, and off we flew to Las Vegas!

Pattie's sister, Mary, and her husband, Tom, live just outside Tampa, Florida. We stayed with them and visited following each UW bowl game in January. This time, Tom and Mary decided to fly out to Las Vegas and meet us there for the game.

Mary is a nurse and manages several kidney dialysis units in Florida. She was so supportive and such a good friend throughout my diagnosis and treatment. If I didn't know better, I would say that she volunteered to travel with us so she could be there for me, as much as to see the game or spend time with her sister.

What an experience! The Rebels' stadium seats less than forty thousand people, but over thirty thousand UW fans traveled west to the game. We were forced to buy season tickets just to get in! Most University of Wisconsin fans couldn't get tickets and remained outside the stadium in a tailgate and party area, festively set up in a distant parking lot. The Badger band played. The fans roared. The beer flowed. Then the game started.

The weather was hot and uncomfortable. The game was too close for comfort as well! My fifth ranked Badgers almost lost to the unranked and over matched UNLV Rebels, but won in the end on a last minute touchdown.

After the game, Pattie and Mary met some Green Bay Packer fans tailgating in our parking lot. The temperature was well over one hundred degrees, but it didn't bother them! They had a water misting machine and bar set up, complete with stools and tiki style grass umbrellas for shade. Turned out one of the couples there owned a nearby bar called the Rum Runner. Every NFL Sunday, their bar turned into a second Lambeau Field! Since Las Vegas was on mountain time, most televised NFL games started early, at 10 a.m. The bar served breakfast and had door prizes and specials throughout the game, just like back in Wisconsin.

The four of us ate breakfast and watched the Packers beat the Philadelphia Eagles at the Rum Runner the next day. We then played tourist and drove out to Hoover Dam and shopped the Vegas Strip Sunday night. A perfect end to a perfect weekend! Fun with family and friends. Winning football. A safe flight home. I was sore and tired Tuesday, but I had just experienced a truly memorable weekend. And that very day I received more good news. The head of the Blood and Marrow Transplant Department at Mayo Clinic, Dr. Suzanne Hayman, had pulled some strings and convinced my insurance company that collecting my stem cells now was in everyone's best interest. They had approved the procedure! I would head back to Rochester the next Wednesday.

Mayo Stem Cell Harvest

Since time was short and I would not be staying for a transplant, I decided to stay at a new Microtel Inn, two exits from Mayo Clinic. I was expecting to stay for at least one week, so I reserved the first room off the lobby next to the small kitchen area the motel uses for continental breakfasts. That way I could use the microwave and refrigerator next door and eat most of my meals in my room.

I completed most of the mandatory tests during my prior visit, so I was immediately ready to meet with my doctors and get started. By the way, this might be a good time to mention that most of the tests I endured, including a difficult two hour, full body MRI and bone marrow biopsy, were not required by Mayo for my collect and store. The insurance company insisted I undergo these extensive and expensive tests. You know, the same insurance company that then refused to pay for the actual procedure! (Don't get me started on Blue Cross/Blue Shield's illogical and inefficient approach to health care!)

I arrived Wednesday and met with Joan Theurer, RN for the BMT department head, Dr. Hayman for about one hour. Joan was a very pleasant and upbeat professional. She explained my itinerary and described my impending ordeal with confidence and care.

Because of my relatively young age, the plan was to collect enough stem cells for as many as three future transplants. Since a transplant required up to three million stem cells, our goal was to collect at least nine million stem cells.

To achieve this goal, Joan explained I would be given injections of growth factors to stimulate the production of stem cells in my bone marrow. So many cells would be produced they would be forced into the bloodstream, where they could be harvested using an apheresis machine. Joan expected the growth factor to take three or four days to stimulate stem cell production enough to begin the three or four day harvesting process. She cautioned me, both parts of the procedure could take longer. It just depended on the individual.

I had spoken with a number of transplant patients over the past year and knew that collection times varied from person to person. Several members of our support group collected all of their stem cells in as little as two days. Barb Davis in our group collected over nine million cells on her first day! Karl Vollstedt, the seventy-five year old president of our

Stillwater Multiple Myeloma support group, also produced enough cells to stop after two days. I was young and strong, right? Everyone kept telling me so! I listened to Joan explain some patients take much longer to meet their goal, but my assumption was if my friends could finish in one or two days, so could I!

I don't want to get ahead of myself and ruin the suspense, but you may have figured out by now my stem cell harvest was to be far more trying and traumatic than those of my friends.

First on the list was to have a central line surgically implanted into my neck. Intravenous catheters are often used in patients who need repetitive IV treatments and blood draws during their course of treatment. These central lines can be placed in the chest, neck or fore arm. Had I been continuing on with a transplant, I would have had a surgically implanted line in my chest. But a twin catheter in my neck was considered less invasive and easier to put in and remove.

I had the option of getting conventional blood draws, or "sticks" as I call them, along with IV needles in each arm daily until my stem cell harvest was complete. But I was more than happy to endure one day of minor surgery to spare the discomfort of multiple IV needles and sticks for an entire week!

My central lines would be implanted at the hospital across the street. If you are ever told a surgical procedure or test will be "simple" and "only take a few hours," beware! Always bring a good book, a snack and other necessities because you never know how long something like this will really take.

In my case, I checked in at nine a.m. and sat in a hospital room and gown until almost one p.m. I was then finally escorted downstairs. Two hours later, I was sedated and wheeled into the operating room. I didn't think this was going to be any big deal, but wow! Around me swarmed ten doctors and nurses all scurrying about, preparing for the procedure. I couldn't believe all this attention was necessary to insert two tubes in my neck!

Once on the operating table, the anesthesiologist refused to anesthetize me after I let it slip that I was there unaccompanied. "You can't drive after surgery!" he and another nurse exclaimed. "We will have to do a local." "Hold on!" I howled. "I'm not going through this without anesthesia!" I already had an IV line started, and even one of the nurses mentioned a local might not be the best idea.

Was she right! After convincing the staff I would take the clinic shuttle back to my motel after surgery, my anesthesia started and the procedure began. The idea was for me to stay awake. Drowsy, but able to respond to the surgeon if necessary. The only problem was it hurt! I could feel every poke, cut and jab. "You shouldn't be able to feel a thing!" the surgeon said skeptically. What, like I would make this stuff up? I knew that they needed me groggy, but awake. Just one step above unconsciousness. But this was not comfortable. After passing the "Can you feel this?" test, proving to my surgeon I really could feel him forcing the catheter down and through my neck, the anesthesiologist added a push of this and a touch of that and things improved.

Ten minutes later, there I lay with a new set of three inch long red and blue color coded tubes hanging from the right side of my neck. I couldn't wait to walk through the produce section at the Super Target store near my motel and try to pick up women! I fantasized about meeting a young co-ed while we squeezed tomatoes and she asked to touch my designer colored neck tubes! A real ice breaker and novel pick-up line. Bet she never heard that one before!

It was now almost five p.m. My simple one or two hour procedure had taken eight hours! Tired and frustrated I drove, (yes, drove!) back to the Microtel to rest and get ready for Friday.

Next on the agenda; growth factor and Fragmin belly shots! Friday, seven a.m. Sharp, I reported to the Infusion Therapy Center for three injections. The first was Fragmin, a type of low molecular weight Heparin used to keep my blood thin, given my recent history of pulmonary embolus. Fortunately, I wasn't allergic to Fragmin as I was Lovinox. (Not that I had figured that out yet!) The only adverse reaction to Fragmin I experienced was deep and dark bruising at the injection sites.

The Fragmin was followed by two syringes full of growth factor. And this was all repeated twice daily; once in the morning and once at night.

No one likes shots and needles. Some patients don't seem to mind too much. Others can become hysterical at the sight of a syringe. I fall somewhere in between. In the grand

133

scheme of things, a few needle sticks and pricks are a small price to pay for staying alive! But human beings and their fears and feelings aren't always logical. I remember one of my first thoughts after hearing the word "cancer" was the dread I felt in anticipation of endless blood draws, injections and IV's. Isn't that funny? A person learns he has cancer and he immediately fears being stuck by needles even more than death.

Part of my fear stemmed from a negative experience I had while undergoing knee surgery following my senior high school football season. I had asked to delay the surgery until after the season. My doctor reluctantly agreed. I will never forget lying on the operating table being prepped for surgery. My nurse was having a heck of a time starting my IV. Even sedated, the pain was intense as she ineptly dug around in my hand, searching for an elusive vein. Sensing my discomfort, one of the doctors called for another nurse to complete the task. After several additional attempts, my line was started and the surgery proceeded without incident But my memories of that day over thirty years ago are vivid indeed! Like the smell of freshly baked bread or cookies, pain is unforgetable.

My fear decreased gradually from then on. Initially, I broke into a cold sweat while even thinking about having my blood drawn! The first time I drove down to the Osceola Medical Center for a blood draw after my diagnosis, I circled the block repeatedly before getting up the nerve to park and go inside.

Too late to worry about that now. If I didn't like needles, I was definitely in the wrong place! I endured belly shots before when I was hospitalized in July with my pneumonia and pulmonary embolus. Actually, those injections weren't that big of a deal. Twice daily shots just under the skin. The Fragmin injections were the same type of thing. The bruising looked bad, but the pain was OK. But these growth factor shots were a big deal! Since the medication did not fit into a single syringe, two shots were needed to deliver the prescribed dose. The needle was larger than the one used for Heparin. Worse yet, it took up to ninety seconds for the nurse to empty each syringe. If the nurse pushed too hard or too fast, it would burn big time! Too slow, and the wait became excruciating, in addition to the pain.

Now, if things had gone as expected, this also wouldn't have been a terribly big deal. But after the projected three days of growth factor injections failed to produce the desired results, the transplant nurse decided to up my dose to three shots, twice a day! To make matters worse, my twice daily Fragmin shots continued to leave my stomach bruised and sore. Because Heparin and Fragmin were blood thinners, there was a large black and jaundice yellow bruise about the size of a half dollar at each injection site. Eventually, the bruises all ran together, making it look like I was wearing a black and gold belt around my waist. By the fifth day, my nurse had run out of places to stick the needles, so we invented a new game: find a spot to stick the needle! Looking back, pin the tail on the donkey or playing darts would be much more fun!

Evenings were pretty quiet at Mayo. I was usually scheduled for my second round of growth factor shots around eight p.m. The normally packed waiting room was nearly empty. I dialed a house phone, letting the skeleton crew in back know I was there. The wait was usually short. Most times a nurse I hadn't had before would step out into the waiting room and escort me back to one of the therapy rooms.

On this particular rainy night, the nurse seemed new or, at the very least, uncertain. She didn't even try to hide her horror as I lifted my shirt so that she could try and find an area around my abdomen that wasn't too bruised to inject. Not identifying a suitable area, she decided to reach around my left side almost to my back. Now I'm not sure if it was the location she choose or her inexperience or just bad luck, but as she pushed the needle into my side, I yelped and almost jumped out of my seat! Man that stung! I placed my hand over hers and the syringe. Startled, she declared that she would need to start over in another spot. "No, you won't!" I stated through clenched teeth. "Keep going! Don't stop now!"

We argued for about thirty seconds until she again began to push the growth factor quickly into my back. Better that than starting over and sticking me again! I later learned three or four patients waiting outside were quite alarmed when they heard me scream. I bet they thought twice before letting that nurse go after them with a needle...

I only had the same nurse one other time during my evening sessions at the Infusion Therapy Center. The following night, who walked around the corner to escort me back for my shots but, you guessed it, the nurse from the previous evening! When she saw I was her next patient, I swear she turned white! I think she was more uncomfortable than I was.

It wasn't raining like the night before. But it was overcast and very windy. I was apprehensive to say the least as I settled back into my seat, which looked and felt very similar to a dentist's chair. I reassured her everything would be fine. I'm not sure I believed it myself!

But this time things went OK. As my nurse prepared her syringes, I became surprisingly relaxed. My seat back was very warm, almost hot. It seemed to subtly pulse and vibrate as the nurse pushed all three syringes full of growth factor slowly into my abdomen with very little pain. I was eerily calm. I was warm and moist with sweat from my neck down to my feet. Time seemed to stop. It was truly a peaceful, almost spiritual experience.

As she finished, I thanked her for taking the extra step to select a heated massage chair to help me relax following our traumatic encounter the night before. The nurse looked at me blankly, perplexed. "Your chair isn't heated," she said. "And it certainly doesn't vibrate!" "But didn't you feel it?" I asked. "Didn't you feel the heat, the vibration of the chair seat and back?" I could tell she wasn't comfortable talking about this. But she did mention that, yes, things certainly went better tonight than the night before.

I returned to the lobby wobbly and shaken. What had just happened? Before I left that evening, I walked back to the therapy room to inspect the chair. She was right! No heat, no massage feature at all. I was sure it hadn't been my imagination. I had the warm, damp clothes to prove it!

Do you believe in ghosts? My wife does. I'm not sure if I do or not. But I swear to you, my chair was hot and I felt an overwhelming, supernatural calm and peace that night in room ten of the Infusion Unit at Mayo Clinic.

Following two extra sessions of three growth factor shots each, Tuesday night I received the call I had been waiting for. There were finally enough stem cells circulating in my blood to start apheresis. I was to report Wednesday at seven a.m. to begin my stem cell collection.

The Transfusion Center was located on the tenth floor of the Gondo Building at Mayo. Bright, spacious and well equipped, this state of the art department was impressive indeed! I visited here once before during my August orientation and testing marathon. An enthusiastic supervisor had escorted Pattie and me through the halls where we saw several of the four or six bed clusters of patients connected to large, space age looking equipment called apheresis machines.

There are several different types of apheresis machines, but all work basically the same way. The patient's blood is drawn into the machine where stem cells are collected, then the blood is returned otherwise intact. Each session takes about four or five hours. No pain or discomfort. The apheresis machine is connected to your catheter. You can read, watch TV or rest while the equipment does its job.

The staff at the Transfusion Center was magnificent! All were caring, competent professionals. But one nurse in particular made my daily visits much more tolerable. Monica was usually only scheduled three days a week. But it was my good fortune she was covering for another nurse on vacation during my treatment, and she was charged with my care on all but two of my eight days at the Center.

You can get to know someone pretty well when you spend five hours a day together. Monica was personable but focused. She was just the right mix of careful compassion and companion during the long hours I spent attached to the apheresis machine by the lines in my neck.

Monica monitored my blood levels and collection progress. But more than that, she became a friend. Monica understood I was having a hard time, and she tried to do everything humanly possible to make me comfortable.

She was amused whenever she stopped by and I was trying to conduct real estate business using my cell phone. Or when I asked her to pull the curtains so I could use my "jug of fun"— a large plastic bottle placed nearby since, once hooked up, a patient couldn't leave the bed even to go to the bathroom.

Monica carefully rinsed and cleaned my catheter and changed the dressing daily. My neck was swollen and discolored all around my catheter site. I got the feeling that it was harder for her to perform the task than for me to endure it. I could tell Monica really cared about her patients.

I appreciated the compassionate care I received from all of the nurses in the unit, especially since Pattie was often away. Early on, I had persuaded Pattie it would be best if she stayed home to take care of the house, pets, real estate business and her mother, while I traveled to Rochester alone. This was my choice. She was not happy about it, but did see the wisdom in the plan. After all, I argued, since I wasn't going to proceed with my transplant, there wouldn't be anything there I couldn't handle on my own. So Pattie stayed home and got stuck with all of the day to day duties, and I got "stuck" for real down at Mayo Clinic!

It wasn't easy for Pattie. I knew she wanted to be with me. But we compromised. Pattie visited on weekends, leaving me during the week to finish my collection.

The harvest was taking longer than expected. My sore and bruised stomach continued receiving growth factor and Fragmin injections twice daily, even after I started my harvest. As time went on, my stomach wasn't the only thing sore and bruised. The venous catheter in my neck was painful and oozing, making it difficult to sleep or shower.

Sore belly. Sore neck. And I was so tired! The nurses stressed time and again the apheresis machines weren't contributing to my fatigue. But then my blood work revealed an unusually low red blood cell count and platelet level, which confirmed my feeling something was wrong.

Dr. Hayman concluded my first three days were performed by a newer type of apheresis machine, mistakenly removing too many of the platelets from my blood along with the stem cells. The advantage of the newer machine was it performed the collection more quickly. But in my case, it was not returning all my red blood cells intact. The next day I found myself assigned to a different area in the department, where I was connected to older equipment. It was hoped an older, more reliable machine would work better with my physiology. Of course, that meant my collection time would be extended each day by nearly an hour, but that was OK; I wasn't going anywhere, anyway!

No single part of my stay in Rochester was especially troublesome. It was the sum of all of the inconvenient sticks, pokes and prods, a combination of being away from home, pain meds and a different diet that made my ordeal difficult. Every time I bumped my catheter it was painful. You already know about the shots and fatigue. But additionally, my back and ribs were sore from all the sitting and inactivity. I tried to walk several miles daily, which seemed to help.

What helped the most was seeing Pattie on the weekends! She drove down Saturday mornings and stayed two or three days before heading back. I knew that it was hard on her being home alone and not being in Rochester to help. I could also tell from the look on her face the first time she saw the bruising on my neck and stomach that she was frightened and concerned about me! But she was nothing other than brave and supportive— the ultimate caregiver!

By the second weekend it was obvious something else was wrong. My red blood cell and platelet counts were still low. My daily stem cell collection counts were dropping. And what had been an occasional low grade fever was spiking.

Sunday, Pattie insisted we call the Transplant Center to get me checked out. As my nurse wheeled me up and down and around the dark and deserted halls that were Mayo Clinic on the weekend, I barely held my head up. I certainly wouldn't have been found my way back to the apheresis unit on my own!

With Pattie at my side, the weekend doctor on call ordered some tests and kept me in a treatment room for several hours, while the BMT nurse coordinator scrambled to determine the source of my fever and pale jaundice color.

One of the tests run was a culture of my central lines. Sure enough, a line was infected! Not only that, my stem cell collection count dropped so low I was told I might have to wait several days to continue apheresis. I would begin receiving IV antibiotics twice a day, starting that evening, and my growth factor doses would be increased once again.

You can imagine how discouraged I felt! It seemed like nothing was going right. At least I hadn't experienced many side effects caused by the growth factor injections.

Side effects from growth factor shots vary from patient to patient. We often shared our experiences and compared notes in the hallways and waiting rooms. Some would feel mild to severe bone pain as the newly created stem cells pushed to get out of the bone marrow. Often a low grade fever accompanied the treatments. I never really had any bone pain of note. If I did, I probably wouldn't have known the difference, since I endured bone pain 24/7 anyway! Maybe it would have been better had I experienced more pain, if that caused an increase in stem cell production. Because what should have been a two, three or four day collection process, had now reached six days, with no end in sight!

Fortunately, my stem cell collection count jumped immediately after the growth factor dose was increased for the second time. Three mega syringes of painful, stinging joy twice each day! But at least it was working again.

No matter how badly I felt, I was not going to let it spoil what little time Pattie and I had to spend together. Pattie had insisted she stay until Monday morning, so when she asked if I felt well enough to go out for dinner after my shots and IV, I lied and said yes.

There weren't many restaurants open in Rochester on a Sunday evening after ten p.m., but we did find a "TGI Friday's" on the way back to the Microtel. After the waiter brought our water, I noticed a young boy sitting two tables over, watching me and staring at the tubes in my neck. I smiled and nudged Pattie as I picked up my glass and pretended to drink through my central lines. The boy watched amazed and tugged at his mother's sleeve, trying to get her attention. It was a good thing his family had already finished their meals or I think they would have switched tables!

Two days later, after the eighth day of apheresis, my collection was complete. Just over nine million stem cells packed into a several small storage bags the size of your hand. It was hard to believe that so much time, sweat and pain could fit into containers the size of a small hot water bottle!

I stopped back at the unit to thank Monica and the other nurses and staff the morning before I left. My collection may have been complete, but my ordeal was anything but over. I felt worse than ever. To celebrate the removal of my catheter, I spent the afternoon lying in the sun by the river in the park. I barely had the strength to eat lunch or set out the handy lawn chair I kept with me at all times for just such an occasion. It took me ten minutes just to get up and out of the chair later to try and get a haircut. I wanted to look and feel normal again before I returned home, but my guess is I was at least two shades of pale green when I sat down in the stylist's chair.

The good news was I wouldn't need any more growth factor shots! The bad news was I would continue to get Fragmin injections twice daily, along with antibiotics, which now needed to be administered through a new line in my wrist. Love those needles!

After two additional days of treatment, I met with Dr. Hayman. As I waited in her office, I could barely hold up my head, and fell asleep. Startled, I woke up as she and Joan entered the room.

"You look horrible!" Dr. Hayman exclaimed as she shook her head and pulled up my test results on her computer. "I feel worse!" I mumbled and added, "Why do I feel so bad, doctor?" Dr. Hayman looked up at me, then down at the test results and replied, "Pat, I'm not surprised you feel bad." "Thanks, doc! I bet you say that to all of your transplant patients!" I joked and started to comment about how that kind of diagnosis must be why she gets paid the big bucks.

Dr. Hayman stopped me before I could finish. "No wonder you don't feel good: You're two pints low!" Apparently, my red blood count had crashed and was now even lower than it had been when the order came to switch to a different type of apheresis machine. "I can order a transfusion for you, but that would mean that you would need to stay here an extra day or two." "What happens if I don't get the transfusion?" I asked. "You should start feeling better in a few days," she said. "I will give you some oral antibiotics to take for the next week, just in case part of your problem is a leftover bug from your infected line."

She continued. "Pat, the worst is over now. Your protein counts look good. The Revlimid is working. If things continue to go this well we can drop the dexamethasone in a year or so." Dr. Hayman paused. "Now, let's discuss your vertebrae." She turned her computer screen towards me so I could see the x-rays taken prior to my stem cell harvest. "See that white line?" she asked as she pointed to a line between two discs in my back. "That used to be your twelfth vertebra! It's gone. Disintegrated. Must have happened between your initial diagnosis and the last month or two after your treatments slowed the cancer." I gazed at the computer monitor dazed and amazed. No wonder I was shorter than I had been a few months before!

"Is there any extra pain?" she asked, still marveling over my missing vertebra. "How about your right hip? How does that feel?" she added seriously. "They feel OK," I remarked. "Why, what's wrong with my hip?" Dr. Hayman proceeded to show me the films from several angles of my right femur, up high near the hip joint. "Look at that hole!" she commented. "About the size of a golf ball. And you don't have any pain?" "I always have some orthopedic type bone or joint pain," I said. "But Tylenol usually works OK. I tell people that ask that I'm on perpetual Tylenol. I'm trying to cut back, but for now I'm taking five or six hundred-fifty mg eight hour Tylenol caplets a day."

Like a number of doctors and nurses I had met with over the past six months, Dr Hayman could not believe I wasn't in more pain. (Later, after reading this for the first time, Julie, my editor, suggested that I become a spokesperson for Tylenol!)

Back to reality—I was in pain now! My neck was sore, my belly was black and blue and throbbing, my head hurt and I felt like I needed a two or three week vacation! "But didn't you just spend two fun, filled weeks here in beautiful Rochester, Minnesota?" Dr. Hayman quipped. Joan, who had been quietly listening on the other side of the room, then asked what other types of pain meds I was using. "Nothing else, just Tylenol." I repeated. "I miss ibuprofen!" I added, while letting them know I knew not to use ibuprofen or aspirin while I was taking blood thinners. I used acetaminophen with codeine while I was undergoing my harvest to help with the soreness in my neck from the catheter lines and back from inactivity and the soft bed at the motel. Joan suggested I try oxycodone, since I could use that with or without my regular Tylenol. Dr Hayman agreed. "No need to be in pain if you don't need to be," she said as Joan wrote out a script for her signature.

I then asked Dr. Hayman if my bones would eventually heal. "Well, Pat, you're missing vertebra is not going to grow back. The hole in your femur may partially fill in, but will probably always be there. Same for your missing ribs and holes in some of your other vertebrae. But your existing bones should grow stronger and any minor damage should be repaired with time." She added I should keep getting my Aredia IV every month, and take five hundred mg of calcium and a vitamin D tablet daily.

"And be careful not to take too much Tylenol," she added, seriously. "No more than three grams a day. Any more can damage your liver. And dying from a failing liver is a hard, painful death."

Wow! That was a cheerful and uplifting way to end our meeting. "That's it?" I asked. "That's it!" she replied and asked if I had someone to drive me home. Remembering my operating room conversation with the surgeon two weeks before, I thought about lying, but I didn't have the strength to make anything up. "No, doctor, I will be driving home alone." Dr. Hayman leaned forward in her chair and smiled. "Then rest up tonight and if you feel up to it, it's OK if you drive home in the morning. Pat, the worst is over. You will start feeling better soon."

I sincerely thanked Dr. Hayman and Joan for their help. Dr. Hayman may have been an important department head from the world renowned Mayo Clinic, but I was truly touched by her wry wit and easy going, down to earth bedside manner. She was the best!

The next morning I still felt bad, but it didn't matter. It was nice to shower without having to worry about getting the dressing around my catheter or IV line wet. I checked out about nine a.m. and drove the two plus hours back to St. Croix Falls without stopping or incident. It had been sixteen days. Pattie left the office for lunch, and was there as I pulled into our garage and closed the door behind me. I was home!

Author's Note: My myeloma specialist, Dr. Melissa Alsina, at Moffitt Cancer Center in Florida, used 3 million of my cells that I worked so hard to collect, leaving enough stem cells for two additional transplants. Lucky me!

Random Acts of Kindness

Pattie and I relocated to the St Croix River Valley from the northwoods of Wisconsin in January of 2003. We grew to love this area during the past five years for so many reasons. The natural beauty of the St. Croix River and the rolling, wooded hills surround it. The surprisingly rugged bluffs overlooking the river from the nearby Wisconsin and Minnesota Interstate Parks. The National Scenic Riverway, a park running up and down both sides of the river for many miles. The proximity to Minnesota's Twin Cities—just close enough to take advantage of the airport, shopping and sporting events without having to fight the traffic and congestion every day.

But the best and greatest thing about our area is the people. Pattie and I didn't have children. We have always worked a lot, so we didn't do much socially. We took care of our home and animals, and tried to spend as much time together as we could. So following my initial diagnosis, you can imagine my surprise as cards and letters of support came flooding in!

I was deeply touched again and again as people from work and our community, even ones who barely knew me, volunteered their care and support.

It's those little things, the random acts of kindness, I remember most from my ordeal. Random acts of kindness. The phrase brings to mind a good friend and client, Jacquie Berglund, from Minneapolis. Jacquie and her sister, Tracey, created and market a micro-brewed beer named Finnegans. Their recipe is tasty and authentically Irish. Jacquie's marketing slogan is "Practice random pints of kindness!" referring to the fact one hundred percent of Finnegans' profits go to local charities.

One of Jacquie's dreams was to find a special place for a family retreat. To build a lake shore log home where she and her sister could write and reflect. Jacquie and I first met after she called about a lake front parcel of land I listed and advertised for sale in the fall of 2007. We met at our office and began spending hours driving and looking at properties. I shared my recent diagnosis and fight to regain my bearings. I told her of my joy at simply being able to spend an autumn afternoon walking along a lake, helping her crystallize her vision. Jacquie listened and laughed. She went out of her way to make me feel comfortable. As we headed back to my real estate office, I confided I had changed and simplified some of my goals. And dreams? Staying alive was my dream! Now, just a lovely fall day seemed dream enough. She didn't say anything at the time, but the following weekend, at the end of our second (of many) outings, Jacquie told me she couldn't stop thinking about what I had said the week before. She was disturbed and a bit concerned. "Don't ever give up on your dreams!" Jacquie exclaimed. "You have so much energy, even now. Look at how you are helping me. Isn't this what you did before you had cancer?" I nodded affirmatively. "Don't let cancer change your life!" Jacquie insisted. "Don't let cancer win!"

Jacquie's sincerity struck a chord with me. I thought a lot about what she said, and she was right! Living for the moment is important. So are realistic expectations. But without goals and dreams, really, what do we have?

Jacquie also inspired me with her charitable business plan for Finnegans Beer. Like Jacquie, Pattie and I decided to donate one hundred percent of the profits from this book to groups that help fight cancer.

Random acts of kindness. Fellow survivor and Realtor Todd Kohs' relentless help getting me accepted as a patient at Mayo Clinic, even though we only met once or twice before. Opening a card from our company book keeper, Sandy Johnson, and finding a check to help cover my day to day expenses when I needed it most, just before starting treatment. Lisa, the girlfriend of my college roommate and best friend, Tim Hanna, calling friends and family to surprise me with tickets to a Green Bay Packers game at Lambeau Field during Brett Farve's final season. My sister-in-law Mary's offer to fly from Florida to Minnesota every weekend during my then scheduled transplant. My former store manager, Jane King—also from Florida—offering to do the same, even though we hadn't spoken for almost a year. Our friend Evie Miller's juicing tips. Judy Dittrich and Judy Minke's cheerful affirmations. Nancy Fritsche's tireless help and support at the office. Karen Wong's spiritual and nutritional advice. Dan Hames surprise visit to my hospital room in July. My partner, Bruce Jesse, covering for me at the office. His wife, Susan, and son, Eric, helping me keep my spirits up, or moving furniture at our home when I wasn't able to lift or drive. Polk County Surveying owners Wayne and Karl, who considerately worked with many of my real estate clients while I was unable to work. Jim Casterton and his two sons for volunteering to mow our lawn last summer. Michele's pep talks. The unexpected and heartfelt e-mails that we received from business associates, family and friends. Don and Ardis Wright's patience while working with me and other recently diagnosed "newbies," as they explained what our different blood and protein counts meant, and why they were important. The unconditional love and friendship shared with us by Gene and Eunice Early, Karl and Lorrain Vollstedt and all of the past and present support group members that still meet monthly in Stillwater, Minnesota.

All of these people, and many others, whether they are mentioned here or not, deserve my gratitude and thanks. Their love, support and friendship almost make it worth mhaving cancer. Almost!

My Bones

I believe anyone fighting a serious disease lives and experiences life in a multi-dimensional way. There are layers of treatment options, and layers of pain. Different issues at different times become priorities. You are fighting your disease, but still trying to live your life the best you can.

I center my writing around the biochemical process of tracking and fighting multiple myeloma. Blood counts, protein markers, M-spikes, bone marrow biopsies, chemotherapy regimens. But the damage to my bones and that discomfort is always with me. You just learn to compartmentalize the pain. To focus on what is beyond. It becomes part of your day-to-day life. Even though you know the pain is there, you deal with it, manage it, live with it.

I am fortunate to manage my pain by moderating activity, stretching, doing physical therapy and taking acetaminophen. Lots and lots of acetaminophen! Earlier, I described it as being on "perpetual Tylenol." I take two eight hour, six hundred-fifty mg caplets in the morning before a hot shower, two more mid-afternoon, and one or two at bedtime. If I need additional pain relief, Dr. Hayman's oxycodone usually does the trick.

But every day I live in fear that the pain may get worse. Sometimes it does. My lower back pain comes and goes. My back gets tight like so many other people's do, with or without cancer. Surprisingly, my now missing T-12 thoracic vertebra has not added to the discomfort.

However, the damage to my spine at the base of my neck is serious and irreversible. Further aggravated by extensive radiation therapy, the area is painful and inflexible. Even more serious is the nerve compression there. One of the primary reasons I take so much Tylenol is to lessen daily headaches caused by that damage. Worse yet, I suffer from neuropathy, or tingling in my jaw, neck and arms. Sometimes I get "stingers" that shoot down my arms or torso. These symptoms appear several hours after exercising, lifting any object heavier than a phone book, sleeping in the wrong position, or sometimes for no apparent reason at all.

All these symptoms are intensified by cold. When my back and shoulders get chilled, it is as if the capillaries freeze. When I lift or stretch, it feels like ice breaking up— chunks of splintered ice grinding between my muscles. Some winter days I swear I can hear them crackle and pop!

But it could be so much worse! My friend, Gerry, from our support group has severe spinal damage suffered prior to his diagnosis and subsequent transplant in 2007. Gerry is four inches shorter than when his ordeal began. He cannot straighten up when he walks and is in constant, debilitating pain. I need perpetual Tylenol. Gerry's painkilling baseline is massive doses of oxycodone, along with other narcotics.

By summer 2008, my bone strength and pain level have improved substantially. I have been able to increase the types and intensity of my exercise and daily activities. Some days I can rake and do yard work and projects around the house. I can carefully do sit-ups and walk. It is still difficult to sit and read or work for than an hour at a time.

Throughout it all, there still is pain. The neck pain, headaches and "stingers" have gotten worse. I fear someday I may fall, move in the wrong way or simply wake up suffering from more serious chronic pain, or even paralysis. And, like clockwork, here comes winter! I feel my back stiffen and begin to crack and grind as the temperature drops.

Minor aches or major pains. Each is a daily reminder all is not well with me and the world. I still have cancer—incurable cancer.

Back to Mayo Before the Holidays

Low red and white blood counts became problematic for me as a side effect of Chemotherapy. The program was supposed to be twenty-one days on and seven days off. But my blood counts did not recover fast enough to continue this optimal dosing schedule.

Initially, I began to take two or three weeks off between cycles. Still, I was not able to get my white blood or neutrophil count up. A normal white count reading should be above four. Anything under two is considered high risk for infection. Sometimes my count would be less than one during a dosing cycle. My red counts were running low as well, although Dr. Anderson didn't seem to think this was as serious as the low white cell and neutrophil counts. I would fight the fatigue, exercising daily and working part days throughout. But considering what some cancer patients go through, it was hard for me to complain! I was certainly feeling better than when I left Mayo in late September!

Now it was time to address another lingering medical issue. Following my initial treatment with radiation and dexamethasone, I lost almost twenty pounds in one month. Unfortunately, most of my weight loss was muscle mass. How strange to look in the mirror after a shower and see my then skinny legs. And I had no butt! It was gone! All of the muscle had waisted away. On a more serious note, apparently, this sudden and dramatic muscle wasting had so weakened my lower abdominal walls I was left with a double inguinal hernia. This was no big deal at first, since my lifting and activity level were limited. But as I began to rehabilitate and increase the intensity of my exercise, these hernias became more painful and restrictive.

I had met with a surgeon at Osceola Medical Center in July to discuss repair. I had read some physicians were now performing hernia operations endoscopically, using a scope and several smaller incisions to complete the repair. This surgeon had tried the procedure, but felt more comfortable using conventional methods by making a single incision and repairing each hernia manually, one at a time. I would have one side repaired, and then return four to six weeks later for the second surgery. Nice guy, but juggling my chemotherapy and blood thinning medications didn't make this a very appealing option.

I had a similar hernia repaired surgically about ten years earlier, and it was sore for weeks. The procedure obviously didn't work well, since I now faced additional surgery in the same location. I could deal with the pain, but hated to further delay rehabilitation over a period of several months.

I needed to replace lost muscle mass for strength and stability to help complete day-to-day activities. Getting my hernias fixed would allow me to lift more weight and exercise more vigorously. But I wasn't looking forward to the lengthy delay needed to completely recover from both surgeries.

Mayo Clinic to the rescue! While visiting Mayo in September, I met Dr. David Farley and his staff. An experienced and well regarded surgeon, Dr. Farley had suggested an endoscopic bilateral inguinal hernia procedure, repairing both sides at the same time. Better yet, Dr. Farley promised I would be as good as new in about ten days!

My body wasn't up to surgery immediately following my stem cell harvest. But as I began to settle into a routine at home, I felt well enough to schedule.

My surgery was to take place at St Mary's Hospital in Rochester, a short mile or so from the Mayo Clinic campus. Even though I had never been to St Mary's before, as I was checking in I recognized several nurses and staff members. One even stopped to say hello. Scary, but it felt like I was home.

Next to everything else during the past year, my surgery was a snap! My IV placement was the best ever. The medical staff was friendly and professional. The surgery was on time and my short recovery was on schedule. Pattie drove me home that night, and I was resting comfortably (with the help of my new friend Tylenol plus codeine!) in my own bed by nine p.m.

The next day was Thanksgiving. I was sore, but felt well enough to help cook turkey dinner that afternoon. I was off the pain meds by Monday. Best of all, the repairs worked. I was soon able to walk, ride the exercycle and lift light weights without too much discomfort.

It was truly a special December! I could continue to rehabilitate, reflect on the past eight months and try to prepare for what lay ahead. One thing was clear. My life would never be the same again.

Reactions From Family
and Friends

I am fascinated by the different reactions to my cancer from family and friends. You can never predict how someone will respond.

I have already shared with you how helpful and supportive Pattie was throughout my ordeal. From the moment when I first heard the word "cancer" from Dr. Truhlsen, and felt Pattie's steady, calming hand on the middle of my back, she never wavered or broke down. I knew she was scared. But she never showed it.

Her reaction surprised me. With all she went through herself, it would have been OK for her to worry or cry or lose her bearings. But when it came time to help me face my own serious and personal assault, Pattie stood much taller than her 5'3" frame!

Similarly, my father's reaction surprised me. My father had always been strong, quiet and reliable.

After he remarried and I was attending the University of Wisconsin, my mother became seriously ill. The day-to-day details were my responsibility. But Dad was always there to help. When my mother died, he helped me settle her small estate and keep things organized.

My father is as tall as Pattie is short. Almost 6'3", Dad was unemotional by temperament and training. A retired patent and trademark attorney, he was organized, deliberate and stoic. And he could be formidable if challenged. My father was the type of guy who would write three formal letters to the insurance company over a twenty one-dollar discrepancy in his bill.

When Pattie was diagnosed with cervical and uterine cancer, Dad was there to help in his solid, steady way, sending me article after article referencing Pattie's cancer and helping with insurance issues. My father always seemed invulnerable to me — timeless and steady. He didn't retire until he was seventy five-years old. He was always conscientious about his diet and exercise, long before it was the "in" thing to do. But as he aged and faced prostate cancer and heart problems in later years, vulnerability appeared in his eyes and uncertainty in his voice. I had watched him slowly lose his strength and flexibility. At age eighty-five, why did it surprise me my cancer diagnosis would hit him so hard? How difficult it must be to learn your son or daughter has an incurable disease! But to hear the silence at the other end of the phone. To hear him hesitate. To experience the pain and emotion in his voice was unexpected and unsettling.

As my father aged, Jean, my stepmother of over thirty years, assumed more family responsibilities. Far more emotional than my father, yet ever the optimist.

But like my father, Jean's age and health were catching up to her. Even though she was more than a decade younger, Jean was recovering from a broken hip and a knee replacement. Her concern for my health was real. But I could tell that she was distracted as she worked to recover from her own chronic injuries.

My parents both had health problems. I believed they sensed their own mortality even more acutely through my cancer. Experiencing their pain and angst was the most difficult reaction that I faced, in sharing my prognosis with family or friends.

So what about the rest of my family? My sister, Peg, from Texas was there for me as needed. Peg and I drifted apart over the years. But my ordeal and her support brought us closer together.

The remaining members of my family lived nearby in Illinois. Feeling better physically and emotionally, I wanted an opportunity to reconnect with them at Christmas. I joked with Pattie this would be my "family holiday cancer tour!" An opportunity for me to see them, and let them know everything was OK with me.

Joan and her husband, Tim, were busy raising their three boys Ted, Tim, Jr., and Grant. Like Jean, Joan was a caregiver by nature, and motherhood agreed with her.

Joan's reaction to my diagnosis exceeded my expectations. She would do just about anything to help me if she could. So would Tim.

My stepbrother, John, proved to be a more complicated case. John's wife, Leslie, and their two high school boys Tom and Andy, were the center of his life! John's father had left him when he was very young, leaving him determined to be a better father than his dad. He was. Like my father, John became a patent attorney and partner in a law firm. We were close when we were younger. But because of distance and different family priorities, we drifted apart.

The logistics of scheduling my "family holiday cancer tour" were daunting! More complicated than arranging an overseas presidential summit, everyone was busy with kid's school and sports schedules, work projects and time with friends. I must admit I was taken aback with the difficulty in scheduling. Wasn't my health and cancer everyone else's priority as well? Turns out it was when we all thought I needed a transplant, and everyone saw me as close to death. But now I was experiencing a different reaction from family and friends. I was doing better. Things were no longer so dramatic. Maybe I wasn't going to die (at least today!) after all.

That was a selfish and self centered way to look at things! I knew that, then, and know it now. But part of me felt it to be true. What could be more important than getting together for the holidays? Weren't we all lucky to be alive? In fairness, the difficulty was mainly in coordinating busy family schedules. But I had the distinct feeling my visit was an unwelcome inconvenience for John and Leslie. I wanted to meet and talk with Tom and Andy so they could see I was OK. So they could learn that cancer wasn't necessarily a death sentence. But John seemed uneasy about my visit.

Pattie and I drove down to Rockford on a Friday, met with Joan and her family Saturday, then arranged to meet John, Leslie, Tom and Andy half-way between Chicago and Rockford in Elgin, Illinois.

I insisted Leslie and the boys come along. Tom and Andy both played high school basketball and needed to study on Sundays, but it was important we see each other. We met at a family restaurant for a late lunch. The boys were great! As I anticipated, they had questions about how I felt and what it was like to have cancer. Leslie, as always, was engaging and supportive. But John's reaction was a surprise. Every time I tried to talk about my treatment or prognosis, he changes the subject. He was clearly not comfortable discussing the situation in any detail. Perceiving this, I persevered. (I'm stubborn that way!) "John, I'm feeling better for now, but I may only live for four or five years." "But, Pat, you look good to me!" he exclaimed, lowering his eyes and quickly changing the subject to the football game on the bar's big screen TV. "John, I'm OK with it! You don't need to worry about me or Pattie." I pressed on. "Of course, I hope that I will live longer. But I like to be realistic. There is no cure." John shifted on his chair in uncomfortable silence. "It is hard to find, but I have been doing some research about how someone with Myeloma dies. It doesn't seem so bad. I'm just glad that I am alive today!" I became overwhelmed with emotion. It meant so much for me to see John and his family. It wasn't too long ago I feared I may never get the chance! I finished by repeating, "It is so great to see you, Leslie and the boys!"

Maybe I pushed things too far. But no one else could hear our conversation. I'm not sure John realized at the time why it was so important for me to see them, if only for a few hours on a sunny but cold December afternoon. But John was my brother. I needed him to know how I felt. To see that things would never be the same. To understand that my cancer was real.

Reactions from family and friends. I learned to anticipate the unexpected. You should too. After all, it isn't fair to expect others to react to your cancer as you would. You are living with it. They are just passing through your world, while still absorbed in theirs. As cancer survivors, we are a reminder to others that life is finite. That they, too, can become sick or die. We deal with that reality from the moment we are diagnosed. Others haven't had to (or don't want to!) think about their mortality. Tough stuff! Something for all of us to think about.

BC/AC
My New Normal

I hear it every day. "How are you? How do you feel?" Is someone asking just to ask? Is it a greeting, a pleasantry? Or do they truly want to know about my progress or how I really feel?

Friends and family is one thing. But what about people I have just met or barely know?

I am never sure if someone is asking how I feel in order to be polite, or if they actually want to hear about my condition. At first I responded with an update: my white blood count, new chemotherapy dosages, etc. But I quickly learned such specificity was way too much information! Often I lost track of who knew I had cancer and who didn't. A neighbor or customer might have asked the question and seemed quite startled as I gave an honest, detailed answer. Turned out they didn't even know I was sick!

If I were to give a thoughtful answer to the question "How are you?" or "How do you feel?" I would respond this way: "I feel great, considering that I am AC." In my mind, AC stands for "life after cancer." BC/AC: before cancer and after cancer. I have also heard this called the "new normal." It's true! I accepted a different definition of normal after my diagnosis and initial treatments were complete. I have spoken with a number of cancer survivors who feel the same way. And I have heard it in their answers to the "How are you?" and "How do you feel?" questions all the time. "I just spent three days at University Hospital for a bone marrow biopsy and tests." Or, "My oncologist is going to try a different combination of drugs to see if I can I can get rid of this rash on my face and back." But then they go on to say, "But I feel pretty good! My red blood count is up and I didn't need a transfusion this week." Understand? AC! That is their new normal.

Before we were diagnosed, before we learned we might die, most of us would complain about any number of little aches, pains or inconveniences. But all successful survivors learn any day we are alive is a good day!

My favorite answer to the "How are you?" question now, especially when I think the person asking knows about my cancer is: "It's a good day! I'm alive!" Amen! I'm here today.

Complete Response

You never use the word "remission" when you have multiple myeloma. It is as though you might jinx your good fortune and the cancer will return. Because, after all, it almost always does.

No, you use the acronym CR for complete response. Or VGPR for very good partial response. PR for partial response. So what does all of this alphabet soup mean?

Most newly diagnosed myeloma patients are able to achieve a PR or VGPR response after one or more types of chemotherapy. The common definition of PR is a fifty percent reduction of monoclonal protein found in the blood, or a ninety percent reduction in monoclonal protein found in the urine. Any lesions or soft tissue plasmacytomas should also be reduced in size by at least fifty percent.

As you would guess, VGPR is better. This designates patients who have achieved at least a ninety percent reduction in measurable monoclonal proteins. In other words, cases in which the cancer has responded very well to treatment and is barely detectable, but still present. This is the situation in which more and more patients find themselves. The disease is controlled and almost gone. But it is clear it is still there, lurking in the weeds, so to speak. Waiting to reemerge sometime in the future.

Few multiple myeloma patients ever achieve CR. The simple definition of CR is: no detectable cancer left. A bone marrow biopsy shows a normal five percent or less of plasma cells with no abnormal cells. IgG and IgA are in the normal range. There is no detectable monoclonal protein (zero M-spike) in the blood.

I am one of the lucky few to achieve CR. Isn't that great!? You would think that would be cause for celebration! However, to be considered cured of most cancers you must be in remission, or cancer free, for at least five years. Multiple myeloma patients rarely stay in PR or CR for five years and, if they do, the disease most likely returns in year six or seven.

Multiple myeloma survivors are never considered cured. They can never relax, or stop looking back over their shoulder. My wife battled cervical, uterine and later ovarian cancer. She was diagnosed with ovarian cancer six years after her initial cancer diagnosis and surgery. Just when she started to let down her guard, her cancer was back! But it is unclear whether her cancers were related. It has now been another six years since her last cancer diagnosis. Is it unsettling for her to wait and wonder if the cancer will ever come back? You bet! But there is a very good chance it won't. Statistics tell us she has the same chance of survival as any other woman her age walking down the street. Multiple myeloma is different.

The good news is when myeloma begins to reestablish itself, it usually happens slowly. There is time to react. To try new medications. Undergo a BMT transplant. Visit friends and family. But myeloma is relentless. Eventually the cancer wins and associated complications get you in the end.

This can be viewed in two ways— as an opportunity, or slow, deadly torture! As one of the lucky few, I understand my life expectancy is often no different than someone with a VGPR or PR designation. I simply have more treatment options. And hopefully more time.

Author's Note: Speaking of options, there should be several new treatment options available to us by late 2012. Velcade is now available in a sub-q injection or IV. A similar, new proteasome inhibitor, carfilzomib—manufactured by Onyx Pharmaceuticals—is also close to FDA approval. Not far behind is a dynamite oral drug, similar to Revlimid called pomalidomide. Both of these drugs work by themselves, or in combination with other existing therapies.

In addition, a number of new drugs are on the way which don't work well by themselves, but enhance the effectiveness of Velcade, Revlimid, thalidomide, carfilzomib and pomalidomide. My third book, *New Multiple Myeloma Therapies from a Patient's Perspective*, provides comprehensive insight into these and a number of other new, experimental drugs and vaccines.

Time

Killing time. I can't wait! Nothing but time. I've got too much time on my hands. I can't wait until spring! I can't wait until I graduate, start my new job, can afford to buy a car, a house, take a vacation, retire.

One year after my diagnosis, my chemotherapy was working, my complications and setbacks were subsiding, and my bones were healing. I was feeling better every day, thankful to be working part-time and living a normal life.

Pattie and I met our friends Michele, and Ed, for Friday night fish fry. Ed was recently retired, and talking about a friend who was counting the days until his own retirement. Other friends of Michele's also couldn't wait for retirement so they could move to Arizona and leave the Minnesota cold.

They, too, were counting the days, spending time in jobs that they didn't like, in a place that didn't want to be.

We often talked about such things. The winters here got long, and it could be difficult to stay active when roads and sidewalks were covered with ice or snow. Michele suffered from acute fibromyalgia, and cold, damp weather was especially hard on her. I understood! For the first time, I was concerned about slipping while on a walk, or injuring my weakened bones while shoveling snow. And warmer weather would surely help my bones feel better, right?

As our conversation wound back to Michele's friends, I asked how long it would be until they could retire. "Twelve long years," she replied wistfully. Twelve years? IF ONLY I COULD LIVE FOR TWELVE YEARS! My mind raced back along my life's timeline. How many hours, days or weeks had I wasted over the years? If I could only have some of that time back!

Steve Pyle, a retired Northwest Airlines pilot and real estate client of mine would often say, "Life is what happens while you are making other plans!" Think about the time the young waste, that we ALL waste waiting for things to change or get better. This late winter evening was a real turning point in my life. I had always lived and dreamed in the future tense. Striving for goals that were ever changing and might never be reached. It was time. Time for me to change. Time for me to start living in the present. Things might get better for me, or they might not. My energy level might rise, my pain might subside. Or it might not. But I was going to change. Time was too short. Too precious.

Faced with a finite and dramatic diagnosis like I had, my initial reaction was to want to step back, relax and enjoy life. You know, take the stereotypical trip around the world. Or do the clichéd bucket list. What hadn't I done? What hadn't I seen? What was important? For me and for Pattie. For my friends and family. What were my priorities? If I had one, two, three years to live, how would I spend that time? How would you spend the time?

Hold on here! Sometimes we don't really have a choice. It's not like I could quit my job and take a cruise and travel the world. I had responsibilities. I needed to take care of our house, my wife, our dogs and cats.

True, I couldn't work as long or hard as I once could. I had good days and bad. My bone pain limited my activities. My chemotherapy could leave me feeling tired and anemic. But I needed to use my mind. I needed to be productive, even if only for a few hours each day.

About those priorities. I was facing the real possibility I might not live for an extended period of time. How would I spend my last days and years? I needed to be useful, helpful, relevant. As I left the restaurant that evening and talked with Pattie on the drive home, my thoughts and focus became clear.

I wanted to write. I wanted to dedicate my life to helping others who might benefit from my experiences. I would help other, newly diagnosed patients confront and adapt to their own AC, their new life after cancer. We hugged and cried. I sat down at our computer and started my outline for this book that very night.

When a Friend Dies

Most of us have lost friends or family to cancer. My adoptive mother, Jeanne Killingsworth, died of lung cancer when I was twenty-two. But as a cancer survivor, it was difficult and painful in a different way the first time someone I knew died from the type of cancer I had— from multiple myeloma.

I experienced this just over one year after my initial diagnosis. Ken, a member of my myeloma support group, suffered kidney failure and needed hospice care. He died shortly thereafter.

I did not know Ken well. We talked after meetings several times, but never spent any time together outside our group. I do know he persevered for ten years after his diagnosis, despite undergoing a transplant and five years of intensive thalidomide chemotherapy. Ken's treatments left him with little or no feeling in his feet and hands. I could see in his face and eyes the permanent damage caused by years of battling his cancer and the drugs he took to fight it. Yet Ken was always pleasant, always positive.

I did not attend Ken's funeral. I had a number of good excuses not to go. After all, I really didn't know him or his wife well. I had a scheduling conflict with work. It was an hour away. I knew several support group members were going to attend the wake and funeral, so I figured it was OK if I didn't go. But looking back, the real reason I didn't attend was I was afraid. For the first time, I knew someone who had died from multiple myeloma. One day that would be me. Some friends and family would attend my memorial service. Hopefully, some kind words would be said. But a number of others I had helped with cancer might not attend. Because they, too, would have trouble facing the reality that they will die one day of this relentless disease.

Computers

Most patients are diagnosed with multiple myeloma in their sixties or seventies. If you are one of them, I understand you might not be comfortable using a computer. Maybe you use e-mail. Maybe you don't even do that. But if you have myeloma, you need a computer! I know this may not be what you want to hear. It can be stressful and uncomfortable to begin using unfamiliar technology, especially later in life. But a computer may be the most important tool you have in fighting this disease.

This is good news! New, effective chemotherapy advances are being developed so rapidly that using printed material, or even talking with your doctor, will not keep you up to date on the latest advances in myeloma research. These advances are sometimes even ahead of the Internet.

Recently, I went on-line to research a new drug I learned about while listening to a teleconference about new developments in myeloma therapies. I found the presentation to be basic. It barely held my interest. But late in the program, the panel began discussing a new clinical trial using a drug called CC-4047. After the teleconference concluded, I immediately went on-line to learn more about this experimental chemotherapy drug. I tried Google. Nothing. I tried another search engine, Ask.com. No references. Frustrated, I e-mailed several of our knowledgeable support group members in Stillwater. I soon learned CC-4047 was an analog of Revlimid—soon to be named pomalidomide—a new variation, two generations removed from thalidomide. My inquiries further revealed two of our group members not only knew about this cutting edge therapy, but were involved in the country's only sixty patient clinical trial. They were already using the drug!

My point? Many cancer treatments involve drug regimens that have not changed much for years. Ovarian cancer patients are still treated with Taxol. Pancreatic cancer patients are treated in much the same way they were in 1997. But multiple myeloma patients and their doctors can choose from a wide variety of effective drug combinations that are extending life expectancies and improving quality of life.

My friend and fellow survivor, Barb Davis, coined the phrase "Google MD." By using the Internet and keeping current with new developments in myeloma therapy, Barb and our fellow patients, friends and families can become experts in this rapidly changing field. This allows us to take control of our own treatment. To help us build a heath care team and fill in the communication gaps between cooperating physicians and nurses.

Nutrition

The Atkins Diet. The Mediterranean Diet. Vegetarian. Vegan. Omega 3's. High protein. Low protein. Raw diets. High carbohydrates. Low carbohydrates. Organics. Free range beef or chicken. Eat fish, dairy and eggs. Don't eat fish, dairy or eggs. How are any of us supposed to know what to eat?

The challenge is figuring out who to believe and what works best for you! Some people just can't seem to adjust their eating habits, even after a life changing event like being diagnosed with cancer or losing a loved one to cardiovascular disease. But for most, modifying eating habits, while not always easy or fun, is doable.

Let's take a look at some basics. Like many, I have a sweet tooth. Big time! Some say, "Sugar feeds cancer."

There is evidence this may be true. It has something to do with the way many tumors live and grow. The theory goes something like this: As they develop, tumors form their own self contained metabolism, relying on simple sugars to grow. Reducing the amount of sugar available in the bloodstream hinders the cancer's ability to grow. Maintain high levels of simple sugars in the bloodstream, and the cancer flourishes.

The strong message here is any cancer patient should replace simple sugars with complex carbohydrates and lean protein. So I should kiss my chocolate cake and Snickers bars goodbye, right?

Not so fast! At a teleconference sponsored by the Leukemia and Lymphoma Society in early 2008, Dr. S. Vincent Rajkumar, Professor of Medicine at Mayo Clinic in Rochester, stated he believes diet does not have a direct effect on multiple myeloma. A healthy diet is important, Dr. Rajkumar feels, to help the patient fight off infection and help the body repair itself from damage caused by the cancer. A healthy, balanced diet can also help a patient withstand the rigors of treatment. But, according to Dr. Rajkumar, myeloma itself is not influenced by one's diet before or after diagnosis.

Even so, it probably wouldn't hurt for me (and you!) to cut back sugar intake. Let's face it. Sweets are empty calories. For the most part, they should be replaced by fruits and vegetables full of vitamins and antioxidants. White bread and sugary fruit juices should be replaced by whole grains and whole fruit, skins and all.

These dietary changes should be made by all of us, whether we have cancer or not! Most nutrition is common sense. Since cooking food destroys natural enzymes and vitamins, eat more raw nuts and vegetables. Whole oatmeal. Berries and red grapes for their high antioxidant content. Omega 3 oils to replace saturated and trans fats. The list goes on.

Should myeloma patients become vegetarians? Probably not. We need protein to help keep our kidneys and livers healthy. Corticosteroids like dexamethasone and prednisone make it difficult to maintain muscle mass. A protein rich diet and exercise can help slow the loss of muscle while taking these steroids.

After taking Rev/dex on and off for over a year, I was excited when Dr. Anderson and Dr. Zeldenrust decided, since I was doing so well, we could drop the dex from my treatment regimen.

I had been retaining pounds of extra water weight from the beginning of my treatments. I hoped the constant bloating I had around my mid-section and in my face and legs would go away after I stopped taking dex. It didn't improve. I retained water on or off dex. On or off Revlimid. Could it be the Warfarin? I guessed not. The bloating was there, even when I stopped taking Warfarin before and after my surgeries.

So what was causing my water retention? And why wasn't I putting muscle mass back on more quickly? True, I was only lifting light weights and dumbbells. But even though I was starting to feel better much of the time, the muscle in my arms, chest, shoulders and legs was not growing back. Not only that, but I seemed to be hungry all the time. I wasn't underweight, but I still didn't look or feel normal.

I had always believed a person's weight was the most important indicator of a healthy body. Sure, you should eat healthy. But as long as my weight was fine and I was getting enough vitamins, so what if I skipped the hamburger, but had an extra piece of cake or pie? I counted my calories and controlled my weight, no matter what I ate. A simple theory, but it was no longer working for me. My weight was fine, but my body composition was not.

In an attempt to identify and solve the problem, I made an appointment to see a RN and certified naturopath, Leann Ottomeyer, in nearby Forest Lake, Minnesota. After keeping a food diary and discussing the results, Leann told me she believed my water retention was caused by too many carbohydrates. I was eating too much sugar and not enough protein.

Leann suggested I start a low carb Mediterranean diet and monitor the results. Five months later, my muscle size and tone had improved a bit. But the real improvement could be seen almost immediately after I started! Within three days, I lost four pounds of water weight. I looked and felt better in less than a week! Not only that, but my energy level rose and the feeling I was hungry all of the time went away like magic!

I had been eating very little meat, lots of fruit and vegetables and way too many snacks and deserts. Even though

I was eating too much corn and too many carrots (they are very high in carbohydrates) the vegetables I was eating were not the problem. Three or four servings of fruit each day, along with lots of oats, potatoes, granola bars and candy were the problem! These foods were causing my blood sugar to shoot up many times each day. That's why I was hungry so often. That's why I was retaining so much water. Who says what and how you eat doesn't make a difference!

My fourth book, *Living a Longer and Better Life with Cancer,* (Scheduled to be published by mid-2012), takes a closer look at the important role diet can play in helping cancer survivors live longer and better lives. There are many nutritional options and theories. Some make sense. Some are really "out there" and crazy! But all of them can help clarify how nutrition works and what diet will work best for you.

My advice? Read all you can about healthy eating and nutrition. And don't do anything extreme, like starting an all raw diet, or trying to live on wheat grass juice, or bombarding yourself with every dietary supplement on the shelf at your local health food store without consulting at least one nutritional professional. Moderation is the key when it comes to diet and exercise!

Spirituality

Religion and spirituality are similar to nutrition and diet. You know, nutrition for the soul! Just as we can all improve our diets by reading, learning and seeking professional advice, so, too, we can all become more spiritual. Scientific studies teach us prayer and belief in a higher power can improve the healing process. It's a fact!

Now I'm not talking about studies that try to prove a link between healing and intercessory prayer. Intercessory prayer? What the heck is that?

There are studies that try to measure a patient's improvement following intense prayer by unrelated persons. According to the book *Prayer, Faith and Healing,* groups of born again Christians were assigned a patient's name, diagnosis and general condition and asked to pray for their rapid recovery and freedom from complications. The patients didn't know about these prayer groups. Sort of a religious blind taste test.

This is called intercessory prayer. And these studies, first started in 1983, attempt to prove others' prayers can help patients medically. Apparently, there is some statistical evidence this type of thing actually works! But it is a bit "out there" for me. I'm focusing on the positive influence a patient's attitude and/or belief in a higher power can have on overall health and well being.

Common sense (backed up by scientific verification) tells us prayer and meditation help keep a patient positive and focused on recovery. I believe prayer helps take some of the pressure off of us. I'm sick, but it's not my fault! And there is hope! Hope of a miracle, hope of redemption. Hope things can and will get better. This alone can help reduce stress and keep us thinking positively.

Prayer and meditation allows us to live more in the moment. They leave us feeling we have some control over our lives, but without the ultimate responsibility. Setting problems and worries aside helps lower one's blood pressure and anxiety and allows our bodies to heal. Show me a chemotherapy drug that can do that!

Like nutrition, I discuss spirituality and my search for a higher power at length in my fourth book, *Living a Longer & Better with Cancer.* Let me just add I was a bit of a skeptic, or agnostic, prior to my diagnosis. Cancer allowed me to focus on what is important to me. It forced me to think about God and humanity and why we are here, leaving me at peace with myself and the world. How many people would give almost anything to find that kind of peace and focus? That part of my journey has truly been a blessing.

Can Cancer be a Blessing?

Thank God for cancer? You read about it. You see it on TV. Testimonials about how cancer changed someone's life for the better. About how cancer saved his or her life. It can make you want to throw up!

If you have just been told you have cancer, or you are battling through painful surgery or chemotherapy, this isn't what you want to hear! But you know what? For many patients and survivors, it is true!

Let me stop right here and qualify this by admitting it is much easier to feel this way if things are going well. Any struggle can help make you stronger. For some, fighting cancer brings out the best in themselves, their friends and family. Everyone reaches way down deep and finds reserves they didn't know they had. Sometimes this works. Sometimes it doesn't. So far, my experiences (after the first six months or so!) have been mostly positive. My chemotherapy is working. I am eating well, exercising, finding joy and balance in my life.

It doesn't always turn out this way. I often say to others I wouldn't change anything now if I could. It is my life, good and bad. I have accepted my cancer. But would I really feel that way if my chemotherapy wasn't working? If I didn't feel well much of the time?

Guess what? I am going to find out! One thing for sure about multiple myeloma: Until they find a cure, it always comes back! Most likely, complications from this disease will kill me someday. But not today! Developing that kind of strength, enduring symptoms and treatments you never thought you could endure. These victories can leave you feeling strong and independent.

In his entertaining book, *Cancer on $5 a day (Chemo not Included),* comedian and author Robert Schimmel writes about how his oncologist told him to "Embrace the cancer!" There is no turning back. Cancer has become a part of Robert Schimmel's life. It has also become an inescapable part of mine.

Schimmel wrote that getting cancer "makes you want to keep your eye on the ball. Makes you want to define your priorities in a hurry." So true!

For many survivors, that is what they mean when they say their cancer is a blessing. Maybe they didn't eat or exercise as well as they should. Or see the doctor and dentist on a regular basis. Good health is not a priority for most of us until something like this befalls us.

Maybe they weren't focused. Or took their spouse or friends for granted. Or were just traveling through life going through the motions, wasting time and energy on things that weren't really important.

But a cancer diagnosis can change all of that. If we are lucky enough to work through the fear, pain and challenges, we emerge on the other side stronger, more focused, more determined.

The ultimate goal of many religions and most philosophies is to become self actualized. To strive to become a better person and possibly begin to understand one's meaning and purpose in life. Can you think of a more instructive journey in life than being diagnosed, surviving and then learning to live with cancer?

In this way cancer can be a blessing! What else can you name that helps motivate someone to eat better, exercise more, appreciate and better understand the meaning of life and become a more grounded and spiritual person? If patient, friends and family can stay positive and truly subscribe to this type of thinking, it should be good for everyone's health and soul.

Death is inevitable. It is how one lives one's life that is important. Were you kind to others, even when faced with adversity and pain? Did you give back to your community? Did you help others less fortunate than you?

And what about YOU? Were you true to yourself and your feelings? Remember my Realtor friend, Karen Wong, who was diagnosed with multiple myeloma shortly after I was? Karen called me recently to share she is going to sell her home and travel the world! She feels she always lived her life for others: her first husband, friends and family. Now she is going to see the world and begin a journey of self exploration. Karen wants to discover and be true to herself.

Like me, Karen is energized by a new sense of urgency. Life is short, and she doesn't want to waste a minute!

Isn't it fascinating the way different people respond to adversity? More specifically, in this case, how one responds to the brutal truth life on this earth is finite—and time is limited. Some spend more time with family. Like Karen, some travel and search for meaning in their lives. Others try to complete their "bucket list." You know, the list of important things they would like to do or see before they die. I began writing as a way to find myself and help others at the same time.

One thing is certain. Karen is right! Life is short. Don't waste a minute!

Insurance

OK. Let's get real. Good nutrition is important. So is making good and productive use of your time. But if you can't afford good insurance, you're screwed!

As I sit here finishing my book, I can't help but wonder how different my life would be right now without good insurance. Yes, by using all my savings, and with help from parents and friends, I could have afforded enough Revlimid to have achieved at least a very good partial response. But insurance is about choices. Once you achieve a VGPR or CR, do you stop taking your chemo, wait and watch? Do you continue with maintenance therapy? Or, do you continue taking the maximum dose of chemotherapy your body can tolerate? Do you decide to go ahead with a stem cell transplant because your health is good now and you are young and strong? What happens if and when the cancer starts to return? And what about the extra stress while you wait, pray and hope?

Even oncologists who specialize in treating patients with myeloma can't agree on which strategy works best for each patient. With insurance, I have choices. Without it, I would be waiting and watching and not using any medication at this time. Maybe that is fine for now. But what about when it's not— when I am no longer fine?

It is the way of our health care system. If you are rich, no worries! (Well, not as many!) If you are poor and have no assets and little income, there is state assistance and low income help from drug companies and charitable organizations like the Leukemia and Lymphoma Society. But if you are in the middle like most Americans, things can head south in a hurry.

For example, say you have a pre-existing condition. Your insurance rates start to skyrocket. What then? Another insurance company won't take you, so you are forced to pay premiums that rise every six months, as healthy people flee that insurance pool and sign on with less expensive policies.

That is exactly what happened to my wife after her first go-around with cancer. Her rates started to double every three to six months. Eventually her insurance company canceled her policy altogether. Fortunately, the State of Wisconsin offered a government subsidized insurance program for patients with pre-existing conditions who could not get coverage. Although the deductibles and premiums were high, at least Pattie had health insurance when she was diagnosed the second time several years later.

As I sit here finishing my book, it is November 2008. The financial world is in chaos. The stock market is crashing. Credit is non-existent. People's retirement plans are worth half of what they were only a few months ago. I think about what it would be like if there was banking system, no national currency. We could garden, hunt, burn wood for heat. But what would happen to the insurance companies?

I am left to wonder: How would I get Revlimid or other chemotherapy drugs if my insurance policy were canceled or, worse yet, the medical insurance companies failed?

I hope the government would bail them out, of course! Just like it recently bailed out many of the banks and mortgage companies. Maybe that is what it will take to get a more fair, uniform system up and running that doesn't discriminate against patients with pre-existing conditions.

As necessary as they are, you already know from reading about my run-ins with Blue Cross/Blue Shield (or maybe from your own experience) insurance companies are not perfect.

For the most part, insurance companies follow the rules, and most covered bills get paid. And, to be fair, some patients aren't always forthcoming or honest about their insurance coverage. They don't check their bills for mistakes and overcharges. They don't object to tests or medications they know they may not need. Some commit outright fraud by lying about pre-existing conditions. They rationalize that insurance is a right. That insurance companies make billions of dollars and will short change people if they can. So where is the harm in lying on an insurance application or to a physician or employer? Some people feel they don't have a choice. If they don't lie, they are afraid they won't have any insurance coverage at all.

There is little doubt health insurance companies deny claims because they realize few patients will appeal. If you are reading this as a patient, I know you probably don't feel well enough physically or emotionally to deal with billing statements and insurance companies, or the VA, or Medicare.

SNAP OUT OF IT! Try to spend a few minutes each day or so organizing and learning to understand your insurance coverages and bills. Here are a few tips that helped me:

1) Review your policy. Spend an hour or so trying to read and understand the fine print.

2) Meet with your insurance agent. Keep him or her updated. Call with questions, or when you feel you aren't being taken seriously by your health care provider. My agent took the time to meet with me after my initial diagnosis. He helped me understand my policy and successfully fight the company when I was denied coverage for my early chemotherapy and later stem cell harvest.

3)	Enlist your doctor's help. I find it useful to get to know his or her nurse. Be polite and courteous. Develop a relationship. Most health care professionals are in the business because they want to help the patient.

4)	Non-profit groups like *The Patient Advocate Foundation* are often available to help. I have included contact information for a number of these in the resource addendum at the end of my book. If you are age fifty or older, go to www.AARP.org or call:	866-839-0463 and ask to speak with an insurance counselor.

5)	Know the law. What consumer protections are offered by your state? Review your state's insurance protection regulations and options. (See resource addendum)

6)	Don't give up! A recent *Kaiser Family Foundation* study found that over 50% of all denied claims were later paid after the bill was first submitted. Patients that continue to press, even after a second or third denial, are often successful.

7)	Keep good records and be persistent!

You shouldn't have to do all this extra work. It isn't fair! But neither is getting cancer. Do the best you can. That is all any of us can do!

The Future

The future is uncertain. The future is unknown. It is human nature to fear the unknown. But why? Two things can happen. Something bad or something good. Usually both. Why do we focus on the bad things that might happen? What about the possibility something good might happen as well?

My father always said: "Son, the world would be a pretty dull place if we didn't have problems!" Dad taught me to embrace challenges in life. To look at life's problems like a puzzle. Something to be analyzed and solved. I have often shared with friends I don't enjoy doing crossword puzzles or solving riddles, or playing card or board games. No, I enjoy solving real life puzzles and riddles! Figuring household budgets, helping clients find the right property at the right price. Learning to live with cancer. Now these are challenges!

I don't gamble. Not in a casino or at the track. I embrace the ultimate game of chance: life! Life is a gamble. No games, no puzzles, no blackjack for me! Give me a real challenge! I choose life!

You or a loved one may have just been diagnosed with myeloma or some other type of cancer. That is the hand you have been dealt. The challenge is: How are you going to play that hand? Are you going to make the most of each and every day? Are you going to be kind to yourself and others? Are you going to embrace the challenge of life?

Life isn't fair. It isn't fair for anyone. That is one of the unbendable rules. We are all going to die someday. So what are you going to do with each day until then?

For now, there is no cure for multiple myeloma. But as we have seen, life expectancies are increasing, and the future looks brighter. There is hope!

When I was first diagnosed, I asked my radiation oncologist, Dr. Wang, "Doctor, if you had to get cancer, isn't this a pretty good type to get?" Without hesitation, Dr Wang answered, "No. There are several other types of cancer that would be better. Prostate cancer would be one of those. Radiation or surgery and most patients are cured!" That may be true. But if I had to assign a number to multiple myeloma on a scale from one to ten, with one being least dangerous and ten being swift and deadly, I would rate myeloma a two or three.

It could be so much worse! For example, pancreatic cancer is probably a ten. By the time pancreatic cancer is identified and diagnosed, most patients have very little time left. Surgery is difficult. Chemotherapy ineffective.

Multiple myeloma is relentless. But it often responds to a number of different therapies. Doctors at Mayo Clinic feel myeloma may soon be defined as a chronic disease. Manageable over time like hypertension or diabetes.

When I was first diagnosed with cancer, all I asked from God was to feel normal again. To spend quality time with friends and family. I wanted to have some time to live a regular life. I have been granted that and more!

I hope you, or the person you love who has been presented with the challenge of facing multiple myeloma, can someday embrace that challenge. That you can learn to appreciate life and living day to day. Good luck! My thoughts and prayers are with you!

Information & Resources

Here are a number of Internet sites, books, magazines and organizations that I have found helpful. I will be updating *Living with Multiple Myeloma* each and every year. I think we would all appreciate it if you would let me know when you find a useful resource about myeloma for inclusion in the next edition. Please e-mail me at Pat@HelpWithCancer.org with your suggestions and I will be glad to include the contact information on our Website and in our next edition.

International Myeloma Foundation
www.myeloma.org
800-452-2873
E-mail: theIMF@myeloma.org

Multiple Myeloma Research Foundation
www.multiplemyeloma.org
203-229-0464

Leukemia & Lymphoma Society
www.leukemia-lymphoma.org
800-955-4572

Daily online multiple myeloma updates:
www.MultpleMyelomaBlog.com

Help With Cancer. org
www.HelpWithCancer.org
715-271-5047

American Cancer Society
www.cancer.org
800-227-2345

National Cancer Institute
www.cancer.gov

Mayo Clinic Cancer Information
www.mayoclinic.com/health/cancer/CA9999

Myeloma Clinical Trials
www.myelomatrials.org

www.MyMultipleMyeloma.com
An educational site sponsord by Millenium
Pharmaceuticals

Cancer Care, Inc
www.cancercare.org

Neuropathy Association
www.neuropathy.org

OnControl Bone Marrow System Manufactured by
Vidacare Corporation
www.vidacare.com

Patient Advocate Foundation
www.patientadvocate.org
800-532-5274

Weekly multiple myeloma research udates
www.MyelomaNews.com

Access to Online Health Information Sources
Access nationwide data bases for hospitals, local health
departments, Medical schools, state insurance boards, etc.
www.healthguideusa.org

Kaiser Family Foundation
Information about specific state medical
and insurance programs
www.statehealthfacts.kff.org

Foundation for Health Coverage Education
www.coverageforall.org
800-234-1317

Cure Magazine
A free publication featuring cancer updates,
research and education
www.curetoday.com

Renegade Patient: The No-Nonsense, Practical
Guide to Getting the Health Care You Need
BioMed Publishing Group.
Available at MyCancerStore.org

Cancer: 50 Essential Things to Do
Published by Penguin Books
Retail price: $14.00
Available at a discounted price of $11.95
www.HelpWithCancer.org

Stem Cell Transplants from a Patient's Perspective
Mira Publishing, Red Fox Trail Press
Available at <u>MyCancerStore.org</u>

DEFEAT Cancer
BioMed Publishing Group
Available at <u>MyCancerStore.org</u>

New Multiple Myeloma Therapies from a Patient' Perspective
Mira Publishing, Red Fox Trail Press
Available at <u>MyCancerStore.org</u>